FITNESS WITHOUT FEAR

D1596735

FITNESS WITHOUT FEAR

A PRACTICAL GUIDE TO IMPROVING YOUR LIFE THROUGH GOOD MOVEMENT

SARA FLEMING

NEW DEGREE PRESS

FITNESS WITHOUT FEAR

A Practical Guide to Improving Your Life through Good Movement

ISBN   978-1-63676-822-9   *Paperback*

           978-1-63730-220-0   *Kindle Ebook*

           978-1-63730-266-8   *Ebook*

TABLE OF CONTENTS

———

INTRODUCTION: FITNESS WITHOUT FEAR

Many years ago, one of my clients brought her daughter, Megan, to one of my training sessions. Megan was tall for a twelve-year-old: she was almost my height, but stood in front of me, slouched over, staring at the floor. My client explained that her daughter was having a bad week. Apparently, her soccer coach had kicked her off the team. The reason? He didn't think she was any good. He said she was the reason the team wasn't doing well. Having been an awkward teen myself who was more frequently cut than allowed to play, this broke my heart.

That day, I tried to get Megan to join in with the circuit training her mother and friends were doing. She tried, but I could tell she felt awkward and embarrassed. She was not into it. As the women were laughing and talking with one another while they did lunges across the gym and tossed medicine balls back and forth, Megan kept to herself off to one side of the gym and avoided eye contact with everyone. She was clearly a strong child, but she was having trouble executing certain exercises correctly, so I quietly pulled her aside.

"How about we work on your squat?" I asked her.

She paused for a minute, still looking at the floor. When she realized I wasn't making fun of her, she smiled, and we moved into a corner out of the way and out of sight of the rest of the group. While the group continued their workout, we worked on her squat, just the two of us. I realized that she was a lot like me: neither of us were necessarily intuitive about movement, but we both loved learning ways to improve. Because of that, she was easy to teach. Even better: learning gave her confidence.

I worked with Megan throughout the summer. She began to enjoy joining in on her mother's workouts; I thought she would respond well to more of a challenge and decided to teach her basic barbell lifts as well. Together, we discovered that she really liked lifting weights. Soon, I introduced her to "the snatch" and the "clean and jerk," the competitive Olympic lifts. As Megan grew more proficient with barbells, her strength, coordination, and confidence grew. Within a year, I took her to her first weightlifting meet. Over the next three years she went on to compete twice at USA Weightlifting Youth Nationals. The strength and athleticism she developed through weightlifting served her in other areas as well. As a freshman in high school, Megan joined the track and field team and became one of the highest ranked pole vaulters in her state.

Megan exemplified what I've seen with countless individuals who have walked through my gym door.

I have seen time and time again that **when people are given the opportunity to learn, they are often willing to work harder.** They see their accomplishments as the product of their own knowledge and effort and are motivated to continue to learn and push past their preconceived limits.

When my clients recognize that I see them as an individual, they feel safe and supported. They trust that I'm not going to hurt them or ask them to do anything they aren't capable of. Although I know a number of fellow trainers who subscribe to this same philosophy, I see many trainers, gyms, and exercise classes that do not. The emphasis seems to be more on pushing clients to their absolute limit without attention to individual differences and abilities. I see many people give up before they ever really get started; they return to their sedentary life feeling defeated and hopeless.

As much as people might prefer the safety and comfort of their couch, we were not built to be sedentary. Our evolutionary history as hunter-gatherers depended on an active lifestyle but also gifted us with a penchant for high-calorie foods and a tendency to be conservative with energy expenditure whenever possible.[1] Without regular physical activity, we are at much higher risk for a number of health problems that not only limit our lifespan but also limit our abilities and quality of life while we're still living.

---

1   Harold H. Lee, Jessica A. Emerson, and David M. Williams, "The Exercise–Affect–Adherence Pathway: An Evolutionary Perspective," *Frontiers in Psychology* 7, article no. 1285 (2016): 3.

One of the non-mysteries in health research is why fewer and fewer people are exercising despite the known health benefits. People are living longer due to medical interventions, but that doesn't necessarily mean a better quality of life. More people are living with chronic diseases associated with inactivity than ever before. Cardiovascular disease, diabetes, obesity, arthritis, etc. are crippling but not necessarily killing a portion of our population.[2]

Our longevity is not coupled with wellness. The health benefits of even small amounts of increased physical activity are staggeringly positive, and yet, the number of people actively exercising continues to decline while sedentary behaviors increase.[3] The reason for this? In part it is because most people don't find exercise pleasant and/or don't believe they can exercise enough to make a difference.[4]

I believe that a big part of the problem with getting people to exercise is a perception problem. And a big part of that problem is the fitness industry itself.

2   Eileen M Crimmins and Hiram Beltrán-Sánchez, "Mortality and Morbidity Trends: Is There Compression of Morbidity?" *The Journals of Gerontology. Series B, Psychological Sciences and Social Sciences* 66, no. 1 (January 2011): 76–79.

3   Kenneth E. Powell, Amanda E. Paluch, and Steven N. Blair, "Physical Activity for Health: What Kind? How Much? How Intense? On Top of What?" *Annual Review of Public Health* 32, no. 1 (March 18, 2011): 350-351.; Margie E Lachman et al., "When Adults Don't Exercise: Behavioral Strategies to Increase Physical Activity in Sedentary Middle-Aged and Older Adults," *Innovation in Aging* 2, no. igy007 (April 5, 2018): 2.

4   Margie E Lachman et al., "When Adults Don't Exercise: Behavioral Strategies to Increase Physical Activity in Sedentary Middle-Aged and Older Adults," *Innovation in Aging* 2, no. igy007 (April 5, 2018): 5.; Lee, Emerson, and Williams, "The Exercise–Affect–Adherence Pathway: An Evolutionary Perspective,": 2.

THE FITNESS INDUSTRY HAS A PROBLEM

Whether in gyms, magazines, fitness classes, or videos, current fitness trends:

- focus on high-intensity workouts that take the exerciser into an all-out effort and keeps them there.
- condition us to think that "No Pain, No Gain" is the only way.
- tend not to teach how to move correctly.
- on the rare occasions when movement training *is* provided, it isn't individualized for different body types, limb lengths, or strengths and weaknesses.
- commonly cause acute and overuse injuries.[5]
- can feel unwelcoming and intimidating to the not-already-fit.
- are extremely unpleasant for those not ready for or used to them.

Is it any wonder why people simply avoid exercise altogether?

THERE IS A BETTER WAY

In my research and practice, I've learned there is an entirely different philosophical approach that one can take with training and exercise that is:

---

5   R. Aicale, D. Tarantino, and N. Maffulli, "Overuse Injuries in Sport: A Comprehensive Overview," *Journal of Orthopaedic Surgery and Research* 13, no. 1, article no. 309 (December 5, 2018): 1-7; Rutgers University. "High-Intensity Interval Training Increases Injuries, Research Shows: White Men Aged 20 to 39 Were Injured Most, Study Finds." *ScienceDaily.* press release, April 9, 2019, on the Science Daily website.

- more effective in the long term
- safe
- inclusive of everyone
- doesn't involve pushing oneself to one's absolute limit every workout

I didn't invent this, and you don't have to take my word for it. The top athletes in the world have taken this same approach to training over the past century. It has won them Olympic medals, World Championships, and World Cups of all kinds. High-level coaches, sports scientists, and exercise physiologists from around the world have been pushing back against the "No Pain, No Gain" philosophy, as they know it has no place in high-level performance training. In what some consider the bible of strength and conditioning, *Supertraining*, authors Mel Siff and Yuri Verkhoshansky make their thoughts on this concept very clear:

"The common belief of 'the more training the better' or 'no gain without pain' has persisted since ancient times, largely as a result of the notion that increasing levels of success demand more work and pain. This often unfortunate principle sometimes continues to be imposed on misguided athletes either by themselves or by uninformed coaches, since they maintain that the optimum training load is the maximum training load a person can endure without injury."

VERKHOSHANSKY AND SIFF, *SUPERTRAINING*[6]

6   Yuri Verkhoshansky and Mel C. Siff, *Supertraining*, Sixth Edition-Expanded Version (Rome: Verkoshansky, 2009): 460.

Here's the secret: while you do have to put in the work, you don't actually have to go hard every session to get the results you want.

Research has shown us that athletes who consistently train using a majority of low-intensity workouts actually perform better in competitions than their "no pain, no gain" compatriots.[7] Why? Because training at lower intensities allows them to be focused on skill development, which results in higher quality movement. Higher quality movement allows them to open the throttle on competition day more easily and more efficiently. This results in better performance.

Training, at its core, is simply a form of physical learning. Like all learning, you can't jump in at an advanced level and expect to perform well. Rather, you need to practice and perfect the basics with diligent, intentional instruction.

WHY ME?

My struggles with fitness began in high school gym class. I was not only out of shape, but I was also terribly uncoordinated and small for my age. But I had dreams of athletic excellence. We didn't have open tryouts for sports teams at my high school. Rather, our PE teacher would introduce us to a week or two of different sports at a time, and if she saw potential, she asked you to sign up for the team tryouts.

---

7   Stephen Seiler and Espen Tonnessen, "Intervals, Thresholds, and Long Slow Distance: The Role of Intensity and Duration in Endurance Training," *Sports Science* 13 (2009): 50-51.

During our introduction to track and field, it was clear I wasn't fast; however, I became especially excited about jumping hurdles. After all, I was light, had long legs and loved to jump. The problem with hurdles is that if you catch your foot on the top as you go over, you not only pull the hurdle over, but you also risk not recovering in time to hit your next stride. My attempts resulted in several spectacular crashes and a few dead-last finishes. Hence, I was never tapped to try out for the team. I can't really blame the coach. I imagine it was frightening to behold. This showed me that my desire to be an athlete just wasn't enough to get me there. I was not fast, or strong. I figured that was my lot in life.

Fortunately, it wasn't.

When I began high school, I spent a lot of time at a local horse farm riding, caring for, and training horses. Despite being small, I found that carrying hay bales and water buckets and cleaning stalls made me quite strong. I also began to learn how to observe movement in both the horses and riders I was training and teaching. *Observation and teaching were the cornerstone of their success. Patience and consistent practice did the rest.*

Even though the purpose of the farm was to train and rehab "lost cause" horses who were deemed untrainable, we were very successful at turning the majority of these horses into competitive show horses and pleasure-riding horses. Clearly, formerly dangerous animals could be turned into top-notch athletes if you were patient and taught them well.

I figured the same must be true for people, but it was difficult to figure out exactly how to do that.

The trainers I worked with, the fitness articles, and books I read did not teach biomechanics and basic programming. The goal of most of the workouts I encountered seemed to be focused mainly on making me tired. Exercises were described in one-size-fits-all cookie cutter versions rather than a description that allowed me, the individual, to learn how to move well based on my strengths, weaknesses, and body differences. This is when I realized that the fitness industry is primarily interested in two things: burning calories and building muscle.

Why is this a problem? Because burning calories and building muscle are actually rather minor side effects of the more comprehensive attributes that good training has to offer. When you only focus on the visual effects that training can have on your body (fat loss and muscle growth), you miss out on ways to train more effectively—ways that will not only deliver the visual effects, but the health benefits, athleticism, and quality of life. If you know how to train correctly, you can have ALL those things while avoiding injury. The best part is you don't have to kill yourself in the gym to accomplish it.

I would not be deterred. I knew I needed to educate myself, so I studied and got certified as a personal trainer. I took in-person certification courses on kettlebell training, barbell training, and even my great nemesis, track and field. I continued to learn as much as I could from not only sports scientists and coaches, but physiologists, neuroscientists, and evolutionary biologists. I began to discern which voices in the fitness industry based their recommendations on science and successful practices as opposed to those who perpetuated unsubstantiated and sometimes dangerous trends.

I put that education into practice training everyday people from every walk of life and became the coach of several athletes in weightlifting and powerlifting who competed in National and World competitions. I also coached youth teams, track and field clubs, cross country, lacrosse, and even ran a strength and conditioning program.

In my own training, I was able to overcome chronic back and hip pain and got much stronger over the years. Eventually, I took up the sport of Highland Games (throwing heavy things in a kilt) at the age of forty and competed at some of the top games in the country. Even though I'd rather sit on the couch than go for a run, I challenged myself by completing a few Warrior Dashes, a Tough Mudder, and a half-marathon.

In a nutshell, that uncoordinated, unathletic kid who couldn't make the track team in high school became a top-notch coach and athlete in her forties.

FITNESS WITHOUT FEAR

In my experience as a trainer and coach, I have found that many people are afraid to take on the challenge of changing their lives because, quite frankly, fitness is scary. Going to the gym often involves hard sales pitches, dozens of torture devices called "exercise machines," and amazing physiques that make us feel like we'll never stack up. If you don't know what to do once you are in the gym, and many people don't, you might join an all-too-common high-intensity workout class that can be rather unpleasant, especially for beginners. Fear of failure or looking stupid prevents many people from going to the gym even when they are aware of the health benefits of exercise.

Many of my clients have come to me because:

- they had a bad experience with a trainer or a commercial gym.
- they are embarrassed to be in a gym not knowing what to do.
- they have a goal they want to reach and just don't know how to get there.
- they don't know if or how they can come back from an injury or damage caused by bad training.
- they are afraid. My clients' fears have included:
  – fear of failure
  – fear of not fitting in
  – fear that it's "too late" for them to get any better
  – literal fear of the sensation of raising their heart rate— it feels like anxiety or a medical issue they have experienced in the past.

So how do I help my clients conquer their fears?

I start by giving them back control.

Time and time again, I have found that people empowered with knowledge and choices feel better about their exercise plans. *I teach them the skills to use their body well and allow them to decide how they are going to use them.*

As a scientist, I know that most things that can be learned can also be taught, but fitness is rarely taught. The exercise physiologist, Stephen Seiler, sums this up best:

"Good intentions to add exercise to a healthy lifestyle have often been derailed by over exuberant fitness instructors, personal trainers, and super fit neighbors who take people from the sofa, to the red zone. And the result is that they often return to the sofa and stay there."[8]

If we are going to get more people training for their health, longevity, and quality of life, we need to remove the fear from fitness. We need to remember:

No Pain, No Gain, is Simply No Way to Train.

I've learned this the hard way. No pain, no gain, is simply no way to train—not if you want fitness to be a permanent part of your life. Once I figured out the right path for myself, I was able to conquer a lot of my own fear and perform far beyond any of my previous expectations.

No matter what your age, no matter how you felt about gym class in school, and no matter where you are with fitness now, you can put exercise back in your life. Lucky for us, we are not doomed by our brain's evolutionary hatred of

---

8   Stephen Seiler, "How 'Normal People' Can Train like the World's Best Endurance Athletes," filmed November 2019 in Arendal, Norway, *TEDx Talk*, 16:04.

excessive movement and preference for donuts and cheese-burgers. Motivation to exercise or even to increase physical activity in one's daily routine has been extensively studied and there are many ways we can rewire that evolutionary hard-wiring that makes us prefer sitting on the couch. I am going to show you how to do that without fear, without pain, and without confusing and conflicting information. You are going to forge your own path, and we are going to begin by figuring out where you are and where you want to go.

CHAPTER 1

WHERE DO WE BEGIN?

———

When I first started training clients over a decade ago, I noticed that almost all my clients had one thing in common: they lacked a basic strength-training foundation. It didn't matter if I was training former athletes, recreational runners, or people who hadn't gotten off the couch since high school gym class—they all seemed to suffer from the same weaknesses and inflexibility that affected their posture, joints, and ability to move well. Though the severity of their conditions varied by different degrees, all my trainees came to me complaining of hip, back, neck pain, poor posture, and poor balance. This was my first clue that there was something seriously wrong here–all those things together are what eventually lead people to sedentary lifestyles and its resulting disability. I knew I had to intervene. But how?

I found all it took was some simple strength training with a focus on good posture and full body movements *that were correct for the individual.* I learned this gentle approach while working with horses and riders many years ago, and it worked just as well for gym-based fitness. It's a rather simple concept really: ***in order to correct movement problems, we*** *simply practice moving correctly.* In a short period of time, this approach would mitigate my clients' pain, improve balance and posture, and improve conditioning.

Over the years, I've seen this teaching approach work with the majority of the athletes and personal training clients who have come through my door. While the adults that I've worked with have seen wild success using these methods, I've found that this particular approach has been especially helpful while coaching and training adolescents.

It's simple, really: I teach skills, and then we practice them together.

A NEW CONCEPT: TEACHING FITNESS

In the fall of 2012, my oldest son was in the fourth grade. It was time for the annual fitness test. It's pretty normal for parents to be asked to volunteer at these events: we come in to time runs, measure jumps, count reps of sit-ups, pull-ups, and jump rope, and measure their flexibility. Unfortunately, the kids in my district only had PE once or twice a week, making it difficult for them to practice or hone these skills before the assessment. While the test was designed to measure fitness, what we were testing was a snapshot of what activities these kids regularly engaged in and, I gotta tell you, I was a bit troubled by what I saw.

While there were definitely some athletes among them, the majority of kids lacked basic fitness. I had to teach a good number of fourth graders how to do a broad jump before I could measure them. More than half of them were unable to jog an eighth of a mile without walking. Half of them didn't know how to jump rope. As much as this surprised me, it also saddened me because it was clear that many of these kids didn't think they could do any better. Like I did many years ago, they just didn't think they were cut out to be athletes. On the last day of fitness testing, I stayed after class and approached the PE teacher. I told her my concerns, and her response was an overwhelmed, "Tell me about it!"

When I told her that I thought these kids could improve on these tests if we trained them to improve some basic strength and movement patterns, she said, "Great! When can you start? How about next week?" She wasn't going to miss an opportunity to do something—and get some help.

Every Monday for about twelve weeks, I taught two classes to the third and fourth graders. We would start with a warmup, then move on to basic strength movements, which we would practice with good posture. This routine required a bit of work, but they enjoyed the challenge, and I interacted with all of them individually to give them encouragement as we went. As a reward, we would finish with some running games or relay races.

I saw posture and coordination improve, I saw consistency develop in their movements, and when I asked them what their feet, backs, and shoulders should look like for each exercise, they could tell me right off the bat. During the last four weeks of our program, I decided that they were ready to learn how to deadlift barbells. We kept the weight light, emphasized good form, and did multiple reps and sets with adequate rest periods. They were pretty excited about this—after all, how many eight- and nine-year-olds get the chance to lift barbells?

On the last day of class, I let them all work up to a heavy deadlift. I had everyone warm up with lighter weights, and then, one by one, each of them went to the bar to lift it one time. If they did it quickly, and with good form, they got to advance to the next round. Everyone lifted at least their own bodyweight.

When class was over, these beaming, triumphant kids had a new word to describe themselves: **Strong**. The physical improvements in posture and movement that I had been observing in them for the past several weeks shone in their newfound confidence.

What I witnessed at the elementary school was that kids don't need to do much to improve their ability to move better. The deadlifts were fun, but the real work was the postural strength they developed early on. Postural strength enabled them to move better. When they can move better, they have more fun, so they keep trying. I find the same thing to be true with adults regardless of their age. Too many folks are put off by what they think is the solution to their lack of fitness, e.g., hard-core boot camps, mean trainers, etc. The actual solution is much gentler and simpler. If they are given the time and education to understand that idea, they can all move forward, and that's a great thing.

WHAT IS MISSING FROM OUR APPROACH TO FITNESS?

I taught the strength class at the elementary school for another four years and the deficit I saw and tried to correct was the same deficit I saw in my adult trainees every day: a lack of physical education.

What I mean by physical education is not just gym class at school.

Physical education is the *skill development* that enables you to move better, perform better, and feel better.

This skill development is what builds your *fitness foundation*.

A fitness foundation is important for everyone regardless of age, and it is what enables you to meet your daily activity requirements for good health.

A fitness foundation includes:

- **basic movement skills**
- **balanced strength in all your joints**
- **aerobic conditioning**

When you lack a fitness foundation, you are likely to have weaknesses that can lead to injury, which can make exercise uncomfortable and unpleasant and put you at a higher risk for disease. Exercise is powerful medicine for the diseases caused by inactivity, but without a fitness foundation, it can be difficult to perform even the minimum recommended daily allowance of exercise for health and well-being.

The *Physical Activity Guidelines for Americans, 2nd edition*, recommends that for better health, better sleep, improved cognition, and better quality of life, you must complete a minimum of thirty minutes of moderate intensity exercise, five days per week. Including full-body strength-training will provide even more benefits.[9]

That amount of exercise is off-putting to a great many people. If you honestly can't stand exercising, guess what? You're not alone.

WE NEEDN'T BE IMPRISONED BY OUR GENETICS

To understand why, outside of sports, play, or necessary work, we humans generally don't find exercise to be a positive experience, we need to learn from our past. I'm not talking our own personal past. I'm talking about our evolution as a species over several millennia.

Evolution is a curious thing. As hunter-gatherers, our genetics adapted over tens of thousands of years to optimize our bodies to that lifestyle. Early humans relied on our endurance abilities and improved ability to store fat relative to other primates in order to travel farther in the pursuit of game. Our ability to walk upright and have free hands enabled us to gather and carry more calorie-dense foods such as tubers and meat back to our family groups. This also allowed us to eat while traveling. These activities required a great deal of physical exertion and endurance, so collectively we evolved

---

9   "Physical Activity Guidelines for Americans," US Department of Health and Human Services, 2018: 56.

to have a relatively high calorie requirement (and therefore crave high-calorie foods) and a tendency to store fat to prevent starvation.[10]

The hunter-gatherer lifestyle was so physically demanding, we adapted to conserve energy whenever possible. Outside of play activities that mimicked the chasing and fleeing behavior necessary for survival (think tag or football), as well as social and reproductive behaviors, we did not unnecessarily exert ourselves. Our bodies evolved to be very active when necessary for food, shelter, etc., but without those pressures, there is a hard-wired tendency to be conservative with physical activity whenever possible.[11]

I guess what I'm saying is that being a bit lazy is actually built into our DNA.

We now live in an environment where high-calorie foods are plentiful. We get our food from the grocery store. We have heating and air conditioning. We drive instead of walk. Many of us have jobs where we sit or stand still most of the day. Visual media, televisions in particular, ensure that most

10   James H. O'Keefe Jr. and Loren Cordain, "Cardiovascular Disease Resulting from a Diet and Lifestyle at Odds with Our Paleolithic Genome: How to Become a 21st-Century Hunter-Gatherer," *Mayo Clinic Proceedings* 79, no. 1 (2004): 103-6.; Herman Pontzer, "The Crown Joules: Energetics, Ecology, and Evolution in Humans and Other Primates," *Evolutionary Anthropology: Issues, News, and Reviews* 26, no. 1 (January 1, 2017): 20.

11   Harold H. Lee, Jessica A. Emerson, and David M. Williams, "The Exercise–Affect–Adherence Pathway: An Evolutionary Perspective," *Frontiers in Psychology* 7, article no. 1285 (2016): 5–7; João P. P. Rosa et al., "Motivational and Evolutionary Aspects of a Physical Exercise Training Program: A Longitudinal Study," *Frontiers in Psychology* 6, article no. 648 (May 18, 2015): 1–9.

of our leisure time is spent sitting as well. Most importantly, we have retained that adaptation of finding physical activity *unnecessary*, distasteful.[12]

The unfortunate dichotomy is that our genetics rely on regular physical activity for optimal health. When standing or walking, we are more alert, our organs function better, and our cognitive function improves.[13] Without those activities, we lose out on the physical adaptations that come with them. Collectively, this is the cause of injury, disability, and disease.[14]

The biggest hurdles most people face in adopting a fitness lifestyle are a lack of confidence and thinking that only higher intensities and durations of exercise are beneficial.[15] If one is unable to dedicate an hour a day to sweating and suffering at the gym due to work/school/family schedules, they may feel it's not worth it to do less. Fortunately, that's not true. Health researchers are beginning to see that even light levels of physical activity provide substantial health benefits.

---

12 Harold H. Lee, Jessica A. Emerson, and David M. Williams, "The Exercise–Affect–Adherence Pathway: An Evolutionary Perspective": 1–8.; Rosa et al., "Motivational and Evolutionary Aspects of a Physical Exercise Training Program: A Longitudinal Study.": 5–8.

13 Shane O'Mara, *In Praise of Walking: The New Science of How We Walk and Why It's Good for Us*, New York: W. W. Norton & Company, 2020: 50.

14 Kenneth E. Powell, Amanda E. Paluch, and Steven N. Blair, "Physical Activity for Health: What Kind? How Much? How Intense? On Top of What?" *Annual Review of Public Health* 32, no. 1 (March 18, 2011): 360.

15 Margie E Lachman et al., "When Adults Don't Exercise: Behavioral Strategies to Increase Physical Activity in Sedentary Middle-Aged and Older Adults," *Innovation in Aging* 2, no. igy007 (April 5, 2018): 5.

To overcome our tendency to avoid exercise, we need to understand the **utility** of the activities we've chosen so that we will continue to incorporate them into our lives.[16] Let's take a look at what fitness really is and why, no matter where you are starting from, it will change your life for the better.

WHAT IS FITNESS?

Fitness is the ability to complete a task. And so, just like that, you have to think of your fitness as task-specific. What are the tasks that you want to be able to accomplish? Do you want to be able to go for a long walk? Do you want to live more independently? Do you want to hike up a mountain? Do you want to be able to play more actively with your kids?

Regardless of the task, there are three qualities that your body needs to have in order to function well in a way that is resistant to injury and does not restrict your participation in daily activities:

- **strength**
- **endurance**
- **cardiovascular or aerobic conditioning**

With these qualities, you are in the admirable position of being able to optimally build a more functional and athletic body. The simple act of building this foundation is going to greatly improve your health and quality of life in ways that you may have a hard time imagining now. It will improve

---

16 Harold H. Lee, Jessica A. Emerson, and David M. Williams, "The Exercise–Affect–Adherence Pathway: An Evolutionary Perspective": 1–8.

general health, alleviate acute and chronic pain, improve posture, and enhance athletic ability.[17]

Trust me, you will be amazed at how much better your life can become.

STRENGTH: ARE YOU STRONG ENOUGH?

Both the regular folks and the higher-level athletes I've trained have all benefitted from strength training. Strength has helped them overcome chronic back and joint pain, regain basic mobility, move better in general, and lead more active lives. Being able to do basic yard work, carry heavy bags and boxes around the house, go for a hike with their kids or grandkids, or simply not be exhausted and in pain at the end of the day are the things that have brought them the most satisfaction and joy.

I don't achieve these results through some crazy complex training system. I simply focus on fixing the number one problem in most people's fitness: *their strength*.

Strength is one of the most powerful tools in the box. It has tremendous benefits for both health and performance; however, most people don't take the time to develop it properly. The truth is that most people from the ages of seven or eight up to and over eighty years old can benefit a great

---

17   Frederick Hatfield, *Fitness: The Complete Guide*, 9th ed. (Carpinteria, CA: International Sports Sciences Association, 2018): 473.

deal from strength training.[18] Strength is the foundation of endurance, power, speed, flexibility, and balance. Without a good strength base, none of those abilities can be optimized.

Strength training is not just about building muscle, it also:

- *strengthens connective tissue*
- *improves bone density*
- *coordinates the nervous system*
- *improves flexibility and range of motion*

Don't make the mistake of thinking that strength is merely a function of the muscular system. In fact, the nervous system is primarily responsible for what we think of as strength, i.e., the ability to exert force.[19] The majority of strength increases in children and people new to fitness are due to improvements in neural coordination, not muscle growth.[20] A more coordinated nervous system is not only better able to recruit larger groups of muscle fibers within a single muscle, it gives us the ability to exert more force, move faster, be more explosive, react quicker, and improve our flexibility. In short, when

18 "Strength Training by Children and Adolescents," Pediatrics 121, no. 4 (April 1, 2008): 835–839.; McLeod et al., "Live Strong and Prosper: The Importance of Skeletal Muscle Strength for Healthy Ageing," *Biogerontology* 17, no. 3 (June 2016): 500–2.

19 Digby G. Sale, "Neural Adaptation to Resistance Training," *Medicine & Science in Sports & Exercise* 20, no. 5 (1988): S142.; Yuri Verkhoshansky and Mel C. Siff, *Supertraining*, Sixth Edition-Expanded Version (Rome: Verkoshansky, 2009): 1.

20 Deok Ju Kim et al., "Effect of an Exercise Program for Posture Correction on Musculoskeletal Pain," *Journal of Physical Therapy Science* 27, no. 6 (June 2015): 1791–4.; Francesco Carini et al., "Posture and Posturology, Anatomical and Physiological Profiles: Overview and Current State of Art," *Acta Bio-Medica : Atenei Parmensis* 88, no. 1 (April 28, 2017): 12–3.

done correctly, improving neural coordination can make us more athletic.[21]

Even if you don't play sports, being "athletic" means you can interact with and react to your environment with increased safety and efficiency. For average adults (like you and me), this means that we can carry our groceries in from the garage without breaking a sweat, pick up our children to play, and even catch ourselves from falling when we trip over a misplaced toy or a root we didn't see.

For most of us, strength is the simple act of maintaining upright posture as gravity pulls us down. Believe it or not, pretty much every activity you engage in while upright on dry land is strength training. The newer you are to fitness, the more strength you build by performing simple tasks such as walking, gardening, carrying objects, and actively standing or sitting with better posture.[22] Poor posture and movement increases wear and tear on joints and increases the risk of injury or joint damage.[23] An increase in strength contributes

21   Timothy Suchomel, Sophia Nimphius, and Michael Stone, "The Importance of Muscular Strength in Athletic Performance," *Sports Medicine* 46 (February 2, 2016).

22   Deok Ju Kim et al., "Effect of an Exercise Program for Posture Correction on Musculoskeletal Pain," *Journal of Physical Therapy Science* 27, no. 6 (June 2015): 1791–4.; Francesco Carini et al., "Posture and Posturology, Anatomical and Physiological Profiles: Overview and Current State of Art," *Acta Bio-Medica : Atenei Parmensis* 88, no. 1 (April 28, 2017): 12–3.

23   Kim et al., "Effect of an Exercise Program for Posture Correction on Musculoskeletal Pain,": 1791–4.; Satoshi Kato et al., "Abdominal Trunk Muscle Weakness and Its Association with Chronic Low Back Pain and Risk of Falling in Older Women," *BMC Musculoskeletal Disorders* 20, no. 273 (June 3, 2019): 2–8.

to one's ability to sustain all kinds of efforts and hold specific postures over time.

Think about the beautiful posture of a professional ballroom dancer. That is what strength looks like.

AEROBIC FITNESS: HOW FIT IS YOUR HEART?
"If you see me running, it's probably because someone is chasing me."

I hear this joke on a regular basis. For me personally, it's not far from the truth. However, I want you to think about aerobic fitness as what it actually is: *the ability of your heart and lungs to deliver oxygen and nutrients to and eliminate carbon dioxide and waste from your muscles and organs.* When we talk about aerobic fitness, we are literally talking about the fitness of your heart, your circulatory system, your lungs, and your cells. Although you can achieve aerobic fitness in many ways, the most common ways are through what we typically call endurance training, e.g., running, walking, biking, swimming, etc.

The cardiovascular adaptations from aerobic training include:

- **increased number of capillaries in the muscle**
- **increased blood volume**
- **lowered blood pressure**
- **increased lung capacity**

It is important to note that lower-intensity, longer-duration aerobic training has been shown to induce significantly higher amounts of capillarization of the muscle than shorter, high-intensity workouts or strength training.[24] Capillarization is the development of more capillaries, or small blood vessels, in the muscle, and it makes delivering nutrients and removing waste easier. At the cellular and metabolic level, we also see some of the same changes we see from strength training, but on a much larger scale. Cells develop an increased capacity to utilize oxygen and get rid of carbon dioxide, buffer lactic acid, and use nutrients more efficiently through an increased number of aerobic enzymes and mitochondria.[25]

In other words, aerobic fitness training enables your body to nourish and clean itself from the inside out, as efficiently as possible.

When your circulatory system is working optimally, everything runs better, you feel better, you think clearly, and you have more energy. You can more effectively deliver oxygen and nutrients to working muscles and organs, and work becomes easier. It can lower your resting heart rate, your blood pressure, and your stress levels. **Most importantly, it makes you less vulnerable to fatigue.**[26]

---

24 I. Mark Olfert et al., "Advances and Challenges in Skeletal Muscle Angio-genesis," *American Journal of Physiology. Heart and Circulatory Physiology* 310, no. 3 (February 1, 2016): H329–30.

25 Hatfield, *Fitness: The Complete Guide*: 108

26 Matthew A Nystoriak and Aruni Bhatnagar, "Cardiovascular Effects and Benefits of Exercise," *Frontiers in Cardiovascular Medicine* 5, no. 135 (September 28, 2018): 1–7.

Aerobic fitness activities are typically lower-intensity, longer-duration activities that allow you to increase your heart rate and keep it there for a sustained period. For beginners, this can be virtually any activity, which is why circuit training is such a powerful tool for general fitness. The most effective way to get the most bang for your buck is to just to get out and do whatever activity you enjoy at an intensity that you can sustain for at least thirty to forty-five minutes, three to five days per week. The benefits of aerobic exercise start with small amounts of exercise and levels off with more than fifty to sixty minutes of activity per day, so there is no need to overdo it.[27]

Don't think of this as exercise, think of it as medicine. Aerobic training not only plays a powerful role in your general health, but it can also help you recover more easily from more intense activities and also help alleviate stress, depression, anxiety, and chronic pain.[28]

ENDURANCE: HOW LONG CAN YOU GO?

All human activities are endurance activities. Your endurance ability relies on both your strength and aerobic conditioning for optimal function.

Endurance describes any repetitive activity done over time. It is often used interchangeably with aerobic or cardiovascular exercise, but it is much more than that, as it is not only

---

27   Nystoriak and Bhatnagar: 5.

28   Carolina Ortigosa Cunha et al., "Is Aerobic Exercise Useful to Manage Chronic Pain?" *Revista Dor* 17 (2016): 61–64.

dependent on the cardiovascular system, but also on the strength of the muscular system. Endurance can be loading boxes on a truck for four hours, walking 100 miles, being able to endure a two-hour wrestling practice, or the ability to maintain one's posture against gravity over the course of a day. You could say that the "endurance" we all require relates back to the concept of fitness being the ability to complete a task. Do you have the endurance to get through your day?

Unless you are training for a specific endurance event (which requires specific training, e.g., running, biking, swimming), the endurance you require for daily living can be developed through general aerobic exercise and strength training.

Instead of thinking of endurance as a way to train, think of endurance as the ability you develop through training to carry out daily tasks and activities as optimally as possible without fatigue.

Many people new to fitness are overwhelmed with thinking about how they are going to get in all the different facets of strength, cardiovascular, and endurance training into their weekly schedule, but you don't have to worry about that.

Any activity you do where you are cognizant of good posture and making your muscles work is going to make you stronger, improve cardiovascular health, and increase your endurance.

The most important part in getting started is recognizing the importance of doing "something," and then doing that something well and on a regular basis.

CHAPTER 2

NO PAIN, NO GAIN?

In the beginning of 2016, I noticed that I just didn't have much energy in the gym or my Highland Games practices. At first, I thought this must be that I was just unmotivated by the winter chill, but I also noticed I was a bit more tired than usual and just didn't have the energy to train and do all the other mom-life things. What I needed was some better aerobic conditioning.

Now, I have to admit something about myself here. I tend to overdo it. Even when a gentle approach is warranted, I go in with all the stops pulled out. I thought running would help, so instead of taking the conservative route by dropping some gym sessions in favor of a little bit of running, I went all in and signed myself up for a half-marathon the following November. My twelve-year-old son, who actually loves running (and clearly got that gene from his father's side of the family) begged me to sign him up as well.

At first, running wasn't too difficult for me. I am relatively strong and well-conditioned. so, I was able to knock out a few miles a couple of times per week right away. I didn't get out of breath, I was able to maintain my posture, and everything felt pretty good. So naturally, I got cocky.

Although I hadn't been running at all since a 12-mile obstacle course race I did four years prior, I decided to increase my volume relatively quickly (mistake number one). Running two miles twice a week quickly became running three miles thrice a week. I also did not dial back my gym-based training or my Highland Games practices (mistake number two). I was initially feeling pretty good due to my increased cardio-vascular fitness, so my weight room and throwing sessions began to last a little longer (mistake number three). My son was having a ball, and although he could run circles around me, we got up together each morning before sunrise to start our daily runs together.

Had I taken the time to reflect on how much work I was actually doing and pay attention to some of my nagging aches and pains, this story might have ended differently. Alas, it did not.

Feet are really cool little machines with many moving parts that absorb stress, exert force, and stretch. Like any machine, however, if you put too much stress on them, they will break. My feet had started to hurt about two months into my running program, and instead of making adjustments, I did the thing that many of us do and pushed through the pain instead. By July, I was forced to realize that my foot pain was not only negatively affecting my running, but also it was affecting my quality of life. Just getting out of bed in the morning and putting my feet on the floor was agonizing.

I went to see my chiropractor, Dr. Alan Ashforth, for my monthly adjustment and decided to confide in him about the pain I was experiencing. As a lifelong runner himself, he understands that athletes sometimes just need to work through their challenges and has always helped me to do that safely. I trust him to look after all my clients, and when he gives me advice, I listen. As I lay there on the table and confessed my training sins, he looked at me as he sometimes does, with a combination of compassion and bemusement.

"You have plantar fasciitis (inflammation of the foot). You need to see a podiatrist."

I wasn't surprised, but I was irritated with myself and a little miffed at being inconvenienced by a self-induced medical problem. He continued with an optimistic smile:

"This is not something an adjustment will help. It is going to take a while to heal. You'll be okay, but it's going to hurt."

He gave me his podiatrist's number, and sheepishly, I agreed to take his advice and made the call that afternoon.

I went to see the podiatrist a few days later, and after a couple of X-rays, a foot scan, and a long talk, I learned that I had plantar fasciitis in both feet, and a massive bone spur on the right heel. In other words, I had overuse injuries in both feet that were going to take months to heal.

Overuse injuries are fairly common and are often simply the result of doing too much, too soon. Our bodies, especially our bone and connective tissues, need time to adapt to new activities or increases in volume. When overuse injuries begin to occur, they start with inflammation, which can be incredibly painful. If you fail to adjust or back off your training, you risk fraying or even tearing the tendons and ligaments that hold our joints together.[29]

Amazingly, the podiatrist did not tell me I had to stop running. Instead, he simply advised that I make some immediate changes to my routine to avoid causing more damage. Sure, my feet would continue to hurt, and they would continue to hurt for a few months, but if I iced my feet, stretched them regularly, got better shoes, and was smarter about how much volume I was adding, they would eventually heal.

So, I got a cortisone shot in my right heel (that felt like it was full of angry bees), ordered some custom orthotics, and two days later, went for a run. I realized that if I wanted to make it to race day with my son, I had to stop lifting and throwing altogether. I iced and stretched and only ran as much as I needed to in order to stay conditioned for the race.

Two months later, I joined my son and husband on the start line of the City of Oaks half-marathon. I crossed the finish line less than three hours later (a full hour after my son finished). My feet were pretty wrecked, but no permanent damage had been done. Still, it was another two months before I could be on my feet for more than thirty minutes without experiencing severe pain. It took me six months before I was mostly back to normal.

---

29 R. Aicale, D. Tarantino, and N. Maffulli, "Overuse Injuries in Sport: A Comprehensive Overview," *Journal of Orthopaedic Surgery and Research* 13, no. 1, article no. 309 (December 5, 2018): 1–7.

"NO PAIN, NO GAIN" IS A LIE

In 2014, high-intensity interval training (HIIT) debuted as the number one worldwide fitness trend in the *American College of Sports Medicine Health and Fitness Journal*. It has held at least a top five spot ever since.[30] This fitness trend focuses primarily on high-intensity workouts that have the exerciser open the throttle all the way and keep it there for the duration of the workout. High-intensity, boot-camp-style classes deliver the sweat-soaked, muscle-straining, exhausting experience that most people associate with a "good workout." Shows like *The Biggest Loser* have helped propagate the idea that exercising to the point of exhaustion is the only way to be successful. This notion is not only false, but it is also responsible for a large number of sports injuries and burnout, especially among people new to fitness.[31]

The problem with these high-intensity workouts is that their primary goal is not skill development, it is the induction of fatigue. Fatigue can be a useful marker during a workout that signals when you need to decrease weight, intensity, or even call it a day. Fatigue is a warning sign that we must pay close attention to as it usually means we may be compromising correct posture and movement and that our coordination is not optimal and can hinder or even reverse good skill development. Understanding how to work with fatigue is important, but it should very rarely be the primary goal of

---

30 Walter R. Thompson, "Worldwide Survey of Fitness Trends for 2018: The CREP Edition," *ACSM's Health & Fitness Journal* 21, no. 6 (2017): 10.

31 Rutgers University, "High-Intensity Interval Training Increases Injuries, Research Shows: White Men Aged 20 to 39 Were Injured Most, Study Finds," *ScienceDaily* press release, April 9, 2019, on the Science Daily website.

a training session. Pushing yourself to the limit in a state of fatigue is a recipe for disaster that can have long-lasting repercussions. More importantly, good coaches and trainers know that this kind of training is unnecessary and has a high risk-to-benefit ratio.

I have had multiple clients throughout the years who didn't consider it a good training session unless they were exhausted when they left my gym and were sore for the next three days. My goal was always to convince them that this routine may be fine for the first two weeks of a new program, but if they were exhausted and sore after every workout, they are likely not getting what they need from their training sessions: skill development. Sports skills are an obvious example of this, but a more subtle example is the fact that I have had countless clients come to my gym not really understanding how to squat correctly, i.e., by using their hips.

What would you say if I told you that it's possible to push your limits in a way that doesn't leave you at death's doorstep after a long workout? You have every right to be skeptical right now but hear me out—by focusing on developing your skills and improving the quality of your workouts, you'll actually see desired results more quickly than you would with painful, high-intensity workouts.

Don't believe me? Let me explain.

If we go back to the training adaptations we discussed in Chapter One, we must remember two things. One is that strength improvements are primarily neurological and based on learning and practicing good technique. When you train to fatigue every workout, your nervous system tends to remember those last suboptimal positions and movements where you aren't fully coordinated. Repeating movements with form that is breaking down only reinforces poor muscle recruitment, bad technique, and puts more wear and tear on joints. Additionally, fatigue has a high recovery cost. It doesn't just affect your muscles, it affects your nervous system.[32] If you aren't adequately recovered when you go into your next training session, your coordination will be sub-optimal, and you won't be getting in the quality work you need to continue to make progress.

The second thing to remember is that for cardiovascular fitness and endurance, the most important factor is the ability to sustain work over time. As with strength training, we want to maintain consistent form to reduce wear and tear on our joints, so we must work at an intensity that allows us to do that for thirty to sixty minutes at a time. Shorter workouts, regardless of intensity, just don't deliver the same benefits.

Many fitness enthusiasts and athletes think that "no pain, no gain" is THE most important aspect of high level fitness and performance. However, when you talk with the coaches who are training the best athletes in the world, you will find that they have a very different opinion. Consequently, they have a very different approach to training.

---

32   Janet L. Taylor et al., "Neural Contributions to Muscle Fatigue: From the Brain to the Muscle and Back Again," *Medicine and Science in Sports and Exercise* 48, no. 11 (November 2016): 2304.; Ben Rattray et al., "Is It Time to Turn Our Attention toward Central Mechanisms for Post-Exertional Recovery Strategies and Performance?" *Frontiers in Physiology* 6, article no. 79 (March 17, 2015): 7–10.

WHAT DO THE EXPERTS THINK?

Stephen Seiler is well known in exercise physiology and world-renowned for his expertise. After twenty-five years of research in exercise physiology and observing the training practices of elite endurance athletes, Seiler has come full-circle from the ideas propagated from his youth in the United States, when he competed in weightlifting and track and field. It wasn't until he moved to Norway in the early 1990s and began studying athletes in the lab that he had a complete reversal of his ideas about his own training and what actually contributed to good performance. Along the way, he had to let go of his American-rooted ideas, the most pervasive of which is the concept of "no pain, no gain."[33]

Seiler explains his "A-ha!" moment regarding training intensity in a *TEDx* talk in November 2019. As Seiler takes the stage, it is apparent that this tall lanky Texan with a relaxed Southern drawl is about to tell you something that's a little bit different from the typical speeches you may hear about fitness. He begins simply with the phrase "no pain, no gain" and pauses for effect. The audience titters with amusement and recognition of the phrase, and then he continues. He describes "no pain, no gain" as an American narrative on training, one he grew up with, but then states his belief that this approach is not only often wrong, but "destructively wrong."[34]

---

33 Stephen Seiler, "How 'Normal People' Can Train like the World's Best Endurance Athletes," filmed November 2019 in Arendal, Norway. *TEDx Talk*, 2:36.

34 Seiler, "How 'Normal People' Can Train like the World's Best Endurance Athletes," 0:20.

In a comprehensive review paper published in 2009, Seiler revealed that over the past several decades of elite-level training for Olympics and World Championships, there was a seemingly paradoxical pattern common to those who were most successful. This pattern was that for the majority of these athletes' training sessions, approximately 80 percent over the course of a week, a month, or a year, was in what he refers to as "the green zone."[35] He describes this green zone as "low intensity, low perceived exertion, relatively comfortable, talking pace."[36] For us recreational athletes and casual exercisers, this is the 50–75 percent of max heart rate zone. You're going to be working, but at an intensity you can maintain for thirty to sixty minutes.

According to Seiler's research, only about 20 percent of elite athletes' training ever went into the "yellow zone" or the "red zone."[37] These zones are described as "high perceived exertion" and "a hard, high-intensity gasping pace," respectively. This is the intensity level of many of those aforementioned high-intensity classes. Seiler's work has shown us that although these kinds of workouts are effective at increasing performance, going there too often actually hinders your

35 Stephen Seiler and Espen Tonnessen, "Intervals, Thresholds, and Long Slow Distance: The Role of Intensity and Duration in Endurance Training," *Sports Science* 13 (2009): 42.

36 Seiler, "How 'Normal People' Can Train like the World's Best Endurance Athletes," 8:40.

37 Seiler and Tonnessen, "Intervals, Thresholds, and Long Slow Distance: The Role of Intensity and Duration in Endurance Training," 42.

progress. This conclusion has been demonstrated in elite athletes and recreational exercisers alike.[38]

Seiler would later describe the pattern he observed as "polarized training." Polarized training is simply the division of training between low and high intensities with the bulk of training, roughly 80 percent, being done in the low-intensity zones. This is the complete opposite of what you will find in most commercial gym classes and training programs for recreational exercisers. Polarized training is good for performance not only because it works but also because it reduces the risk of injury and burnout while maximizing recovery. Some higher-intensity work is essential for boosting performance. Too much, and you are tapping into reserves that you need for the higher-quality, lower-intensity work. That is the work that improves fitness the most over time.[39]

In a podcast with strength and conditioning coach Vern Gambetta, Seiler explains how this model applies to recreational exercisers, i.e., just regular folks working out:

"We've seen this when we bring in recreational athletes. They're notorious, the forty-year-olds that are busy and try to get the most out of their training. Every workout has a tendency to be at the red line for forty-five minutes. But the reality is, is they stagnate quickly."[40]

---

38 Seiler and Tonnessen, "Intervals, Thresholds, and Long Slow Distance: The Role of Intensity and Duration in Endurance Training.," 44–49.

39 Vern Gambetta and Stephen Seiler, "*GAINcast* Episode 104: Polarized Training (with Stephen Seiler)," in *Gaincast with Vern Gambetta*, podcast, MP3 audio, 18:59.

40 Ibid., 41:53.

He goes on to explain that when these recreational athletes allowed their training to be manipulated to include more low-intensity days, their measured lab numbers, specifically of lactate, became much more favorable. Simply put, when you are not in good aerobic condition, it takes a lot less effort to stress your body. A rising lactate level is an indicator of that stress and indicates a lower fitness level. These individuals had high initial lactate levels at rest before his intervention, but after replacing some high-intensity days with lower-intensity, longer-duration days, they had much lower lactate levels at rest. Essentially, this switch from high-intensity workouts to lower-intensity workouts made these individuals more fit.[41]

Seiler says it most simply:

> By and large, the biggest part of what makes great athletes great, is the daily grind. You know, they do the basic things really well. They're out there rain or shine, they're doing the work. And so, I think that's still a lesson to be learned for us recreational athletes that…it's still about the basics. There are no shortcuts. And so, if we can find a bit more time, we can enhance the **quality** of that session. Then that's a step in the right direction.[42]

---

41   Ibid., 43:54.

42   Gambetta and Seiler, 54:39.

TOO MUCH, TOO SOON, TOO HARD = SPORTS INJURIES

One of the first gym owners I ever worked for had been a drill sergeant in the Army. He once told me that boot camp is a selection process, not a development process. What this means is that the boot camp training does not build soldiers, it reveals who is fit enough to be a soldier. If you are not fit enough to pass camp, you can't join the Army. He specifically referred to rucking (marching with a weighted pack) as one of the biggest dangers as packs were loaded with more and more weight each week while distances were increased. Recruits who were not conditioned to either the weight or the distance were more likely to drop out or leave due to stress fractures and other injuries.

I have touched a bit on the risk of injuries a couple of times so far, but this is something we really need to talk about. Injuries from training will keep you from continuing your fitness journey. For a lot of people, this happens in the first six months to a year of training, and it is easily preventable. Proper strength training has been shown to be the biggest deterrent to sports injuries, both acute and from overuse.[43]

An acute injury such as an ACL tear can be pretty painful and devastating, but overuse injuries are just as sinister. These injuries to your tendons, ligaments, and even bone, tend to sneak up on you, persist for several months and can be

---

43   Jeppe Bo Lauersen, Thor Einar Andersen, and Lars Bo Andersen, "Strength Training as Superior, Dose-Dependent and Safe Prevention of Acute and Overuse Sports Injuries: A Systematic Review, Qualitative Analysis and Meta-Analysis," *British Journal of Sports Medicine* 52, no. 24 (December 1, 2018): 1560–2.

considerably painful. These injuries include all the "-itises," e.g., tendonitis, bursitis, and plantar fasciitis as well as stress fractures. These structures take a lot longer than the nervous system and muscles to adapt to training stimulus, so inappropriate increases in load, too much volume, inadequate recovery, poor technique, and any kind of big changes from your normal routine are likely to contribute to these injuries. The best approach to avoiding these injuries is to be conservative about making changes to your training plan, both short-term and long-term.[44]

What I have seen happen time and time again with my friends and family is that they will join an intense exercise class or boot camp in an effort to jump start their fitness. For the first three to six months, they are very excited about feeling better and all the new abilities they are developing. The strength and aerobic conditioning they are developing is giving them more energy, helping them sleep better, and reducing their stress. Then suddenly, something gives. Sometimes it's a sudden, acute injury. Sometimes, it's a nagging discomfort that has suddenly turned into debilitating chronic pain. Now, their newfound enthusiasm for exercise is extinguished, and they must either give up altogether or figure out ways to work around it.

This problem stems partly from poor class designs that use fatigue as the primary goal. It also stems from instructors telling participants to "know their limit" and take responsibility for their level of exertion. Instead, instructors should

---

44 Aicale, Tarantino, and Maffulli, "Overuse Injuries in Sport: A Comprehensive Overview," 1–7.

understand how to responsibly scale exercises appropriately and not let new participants jump into workouts with advanced techniques. Like the military boot camp, these classes essentially become about selection rather than development. Either you are fit enough to stick it out, or you're not. This is not how we should be teaching fitness.

Learning to develop a comprehensive fitness base will not only improve your health and quality of life, but it will also allow you the freedom to participate in more activities without the risk of injury.

Bottom line, we need to be cognizant of the stress we are putting on our bodies. More importantly, we need to pay attention to how our bodies are responding to that stress. Pain, soreness, excessive fatigue, trouble sleeping, and diminished performance can all be signs that we are doing too much. Remember, we want our bodies to adapt positively to the exercise stresses we are applying. Some soreness and fatigue are to be expected, but when it starts to become an overarching theme in your life, it's time to re-examine what you're doing.

When we are teaching children to read, we don't start them out with *War and Peace*. We teach them from where they are. Do they know their letters? Do they know how to combine letters to make sounds? Do they know any words? The same kind of progression should be used for fitness. Fitness is physical education; physical education is learning and skill development.

To be successful with fitness, we need to put the intensity on the back burner until we reach a level of competence where we can start to challenge ourselves. Once we reach that level of competence, we can introduce more tools to keep making progress. Going forward, we will start to take a look at exactly where we are starting from, and that will form the foundation of your personal fitness journey.

CHAPTER 3

HOW TO TRAIN
LIKE A SCIENTIST

———

My favorite training group to work with, besides kids, are master athletes—the older, the better. If you are over the age of fifty and still relatively competitive in the sport of your choice, it's because you have learned many lessons over the years about what is important, what is not important, and what is just a waste of time. My friend, Arden Cogar, Jr., a world champion Timbersports competitor, told me once that when you're young, you can get away with a lot of stupid training and still improve.

When you're older, it's all about dialing in the minimum effective dose of strength, aerobic fitness, endurance, and skill. You will learn that there is such a thing as "strong enough," that your general fitness level is just as important as your talent, and that good technique and skill are the most important factors for both winning and avoiding injury. The good news is that by regularly assessing our abilities and progress, we can achieve a close approximation of that amount of strength in a much shorter period of time.

This concept of assessment is something that comes very naturally to me from working in a research lab. Problem solving is the number one goal of most researchers, and to solve problems, we have to know what we are working with. It's a pretty simple process when you break it down:

1. Figure out what you already know.
2. Figure out what you want to ask.
3. Identify the tools you need to answer your question.

HOW TO TRAIN LIKE A SCIENTIST: YOUR TRAINING LOG

As a former medical researcher, I happen to think that the most important tool you will have in changing your fitness habits is your training log. What is a training log? I equate it to the lab notebook I was required to keep in the research lab.

In the lab, a lab notebook is a gold mine of information. It contains all the information on your experiments' design, the experiments themselves, the results, and the conclusions you have made from those results. No detail is too small to include. For example:

- What time did you start the experiment?
- What was the temperature of the room?
- What chemicals and in what volumes did you use?
- How long did you let your reaction run?
- How did you measure the results?

- If the experiment failed, why do you think that happened?
- What do you want to change going forward?

The generally accepted rule about lab notebooks is that it should be detailed enough that if you disappeared, someone should be able to come in and replicate your work simply by reading what you have written down. Another benefit of a lab notebook is that you can review your work and determine your successes and failures.

When designing your own training plans, there must always be some degree of discovery and optimization taking place. Keeping track of what works and doesn't work, what causes pain or discomfort, and what you like doing will keep you moving forward. When you run into roadblocks, accurate record keeping will help you navigate them.

To begin, you will start by answering some questions that will appear later in this chapter. These questions will help you assess where you are starting from. As we start adding in different exercises and workouts to your plan, you will not only write down your plan in your log, but also your daily implementation. You will want to record reps, sets, distances, times, etc. You will include data from workouts and from your daily activities. It's kind of a big deal if you spend a few hours gardening or chasing grandchildren around the yard, so be sure to include those things. If you take a rest day, record that as well.

Some people prefer an online training log that they can access from their phone. Others prefer an actual notebook. I have a stack of composition notebooks in my gym from years of training clients and myself. On the next several pages, I am going to ask you some questions, and I'd like you to record the answers in your log.

REMEMBER TO INCLUDE DATA OUTSIDE THE GYM SETTING

Tracking what you do in your workouts is important, but the most important data is more personal. Although our own non-compliance can certainly be to blame for our shortcomings, hidden factors can often make it difficult to achieve our goals. Lack of sleep, schedule changes, family stress, or some underlying pain can all affect our performance. Simply observing the whole picture, not just the narrow focus of individual exercises, can reveal a lot more data that we can use to help you succeed in the long run.

Below you will find a table with some suggestions on what to enter into your training log on a daily, weekly, or monthly basis. On a daily basis, just the nitty gritty of the workout is fine unless something like a stressful day at work or a strained or stiff muscle is overshadowing your workout. On a weekly basis, be sure to check in with well-being, quality of life, and diet or body composition concerns. Again, check in with your stress and pain levels. When these things don't resolve week to week, they need attention.

On a monthly basis, take a broader look at your progress. Are things trending positive? Can you find some areas where you have improved? Do any areas need work? With physical training, some benefits take a few weeks to notice, but if you can sit down and take the time to reflect and review, you may often find reasons to celebrate.

Daily	Weekly	Monthly
Time of Day	Scale weight	What is the overall trend in the areas you are training? (Improvement, no change, decline?)
Exercises, sets, and reps	Overall sense of well-being (are you sore, tired, energetic, sluggish, etc.)	Are body composition changes (or maintenance) on track?
Modifications	How many training sessions were you able to complete?	Overall mood and sense of well-being.
Rest periods	How were sleep and overall stress?	Where are you relative to your goal timeline?
RPE of working sets	How was your diet?	Any changes or adjustments in programming or timeline?
Length of training session	Any chronic soreness or pain?	
Any acute pain during training session?	Any injuries outside the gym?	

One of the most valuable aspects of a good training log is the ability to review your training history and identify the improvements you have made over time. Whether it's a change in the number of pull-ups you can do, the number of miles you can walk or run, or an increase in the weights you're using, identifying improvements over time demonstrates competence. Competence, or the ability to do something successfully, is one of the most powerful motivators for long-term adherence.[45]

---

45   Pedro J. Teixeira et al., "Exercise, Physical Activity, and Self-Determination Theory: A Systematic Review," *The International Journal of Behavioral Nutrition and Physical Activity* 9:78 (June 22, 2012): 27.

HOW TO ASSESS YOURSELF

A critical skill I have carried over from the lab is part of the scientific method: observation. In the lab, observation is our most powerful tool, and it begins with some simple self-reflection. Think about your daily and weekly routines and answer the following questions in your training log:

1. **Are you getting enough sleep?** This depends on age and activity level. A minimum of seven hours a night is a good place to start.[46] A good online resource to check out is SleepFoundation.org.
2. **Are you getting the right number of calories?** Most people don't actually know how many calories they eat in a single day. It has been shown that simply tracking your food using an app such as My Fitness Pal can result in significant weight loss.[47] The best way to start making changes to your diet is to determine your current intake.
3. **Are you eating a diet rich in vitamins and minerals, fresh fruits and vegetables?** Diets rich in fruits and vegetables have been shown to reduce the risk of heart attack, stroke, and some cancers, contribute to eye and digestive health, and help control blood sugar.[48] In general, a minimum of one cup of fruit and one cup of vegetables per day is recommended, and those amounts may increase

---

46 Susan L. Worley, "The Extraordinary Importance of Sleep: The Detrimental Effects of Inadequate Sleep on Health and Public Safety Drive an Explosion of Sleep Research," *P & T: A Peer-Reviewed Journal for Formulary Management* 43, no. 12 (December 2018): 759.

47 Michele L. Patel et al., "Comparing Self-Monitoring Strategies for Weight Loss in a Smartphone App: Randomized Controlled Trial," *JMIR Mhealth Uhealth* 7, no. 2 (February 28, 2019): e12209.

48 Harvard T. H. Chan School of Public Health, "Vegetables and Fruits," *The Nutrition Source*, September 18, 2012.

depending on your age and activity level. For more information on how to incorporate more fruits and vegetables into your diet, check out www.choosemyplate.gov.

4. **Are you finding ways to reduce stress and get along with your family and coworkers?** Stress negatively affects sleep and health. Physical activity can help alleviate stress, but sometimes we need to attack the problem head on and find ways to remove stressful people and situations from our lives.[49] Simply going outside more can reduce stress and impulsivity and improve decision making.[50]

5. **Are you receiving regular medical care? When was your last physical?** While an annual exam may not be necessary for the young and healthy, those of us who are fifty and older and/or experiencing some mental or physical health problems should be checking in with our doctor regularly. At the very least, have a primary health care provider who knows your history and can be contacted if you suffer an acute injury or illness.[51]

6. **Are you getting enough exercise?** Strength training as well as cardiovascular exercise is necessary for everyone,

49 Aaron Kandola et al., "Moving to Beat Anxiety: Epidemiology and Therapeutic Issues with Physical Activity for Anxiety," *Current Psychiatry Reports* 20, no. 8 (July 24, 2018): 63.

50 Meredith A. Repke et al., "How Does Nature Exposure Make People Healthier?: Evidence for the Role of Impulsivity and Expanded Space Perception," *PloS One* 13, no. 8 (August 22, 2018): e0202246.; Meredith S. Berry et al., "Promoting Healthy Decision-Making via Natural Environment Exposure: Initial Evidence and Future Directions," *Frontiers in Psychology* 11, article no. 1682 (July 14, 2020): 2–5.; Sus Sola Corazon et al., "Psycho-Physiological Stress Recovery in Outdoor Nature-Based Interventions: A Systematic Review of the Past Eight Years of Research," *International Journal of Environmental Research and Public Health* 16, no. 10, article no. 1711 (May 16, 2019): 15–17.

51 Harvard Health Publishing, "Why Your Annual Check-up Is Still Important to Your Health," *Harvard Health.*

especially as we age. It doesn't have to be complicated or require a lot of equipment. As we reviewed in Chapter One, 150–300 minutes of physical activity per week is enough to improve health and quality of life.

7. **Are you practicing moderation?** Alcohol, drugs, tobacco, and food can all be catastrophic to our health when used in excess. This subject may be something you want to discuss with your doctor. You can even find an online community to help you answer that question if that option would make you feel more comfortable.

If you answered no to any of these questions, how much change is necessary to start heading in the right direction? Self-awareness will go a long way toward getting you on the right track. Small changes such as adding in a daily walk, getting more sleep, and eating more fruits and vegetables can deliver big benefits.[52]

The key to making big changes in your routine is to choose small, achievable goals that are relatively easy to repeat. For example, instead of trying to change your entire diet all at once, start by having a banana with your breakfast every morning. It has been shown that making small changes over time is more effective for the formation of habits in the long

---

52 Joanne L. Slavin and Beate Lloyd, "Health Benefits of Fruits and Vegetables," *Advances in Nutrition (Bethesda, Md.)* 3, no. 4 (July 1, 2012): 512.; Slavin and Lloyd: 512–513.; Worley, "The Extraordinary Importance of Sleep: The Detrimental Effects of Inadequate Sleep on Health and Public Safety Drive an Explosion of Sleep Research,": 758–9.; Suzanne M Bertisch et al., "Insomnia with Objective Short Sleep Duration and Risk of Incident Cardiovascular Disease and All-Cause Mortality: Sleep Heart Health Study," *Sleep* 41, no. zsy047 (June 1, 2018): 7.

term.[53] Choose one or two actions and work on incorporating them into your daily routine until they become habits.

* * *

Now we need to get a little more specific about your physical fitness. I'd like you to open your training log and write down the answers to these next questions. Feel free to be as detailed as possible. This self-assessment is designed to help you take into account some specific details about how you move in the world. These answers will come into play when we start thinking about what activities we are going to be adding to your program. In Part II of this book, I will show you how we combine learning with ongoing assessment to make your fitness journey as specific for you and therefore as productive as possible.

WHAT DOES YOUR AVERAGE DAY LOOK LIKE?
Think about your average day.

1. How many hours a day do you spend sitting? Standing? Driving?
2. Do you have a physical job that requires a lot of movement and/or lifting and carrying?
3. Do you have a regular weekly schedule or does your activity vary from day to day?

---

53 Benjamin Gardner, Phillippa Lally, and Jane Wardle, "Making Health Habitual: The Psychology of 'habit-Formation' and General Practice," *The British Journal of General Practice: The Journal of the Royal College of General Practitioners* 62, no. 605 (December 2012): 664–66.

4. What physical activities do you regularly engage in? For example, do you walk your dog or take an exercise class?
5. Do you spend a lot of time on social media, playing video games, or watching TV?
6. Do you cook your own meals at home, or do you go out? How often do you eat out?

When my father was a middle school vice principal and realized he was spending too much time sitting in his office, he started wearing a pedometer. He found that by checking in on his teachers in person and retrieving paperwork from the main office himself (which was down a flight of stairs and on the other side of the school), he almost doubled his daily steps. He began walking our dog three miles every day when he got home to destress (which was good for both him and the dog). As a result, he lost his middle-aged pot belly and became almost thirty pounds lighter. Whether you work out in a fully equipped gym or at home with a few free weights, you can tailor your workout plan to accommodate what you have available to you.

DO YOU HAVE ANY CHRONIC INJURIES? ARE YOU IN PAIN AT REST WHEN STANDING OR SITTING? DO ANY MOVEMENTS OR POSITION CHANGES CAUSE YOU PAIN?

Unfortunately, pain and injury can keep us from doing the things we need to do to prevent pain and injury. For example, practicing good posture and regular activity has been shown to reduce pain from arthritis and other causes.[54] Likewise, exercise, especially strength training, has been shown to improve pain in fibromyalgia patients.[55] As I've seen in my own practice, chronic pain can be caused simply from strength imbalances that are easily fixed. However, it is important that you keep track of pain and determine if it is getting better or worse as you go.

Chronic injuries are something you may want to discuss with your doctor. What I'm talking about here are joint injuries, diseases such as arthritis and spinal stenosis, a torn ACL, or a torn rotator cuff. You may have already found some workarounds for these conditions, but it's good to discuss alternative regimens with your doctor or physical therapist. For example, riding a bike or using an elliptical may be a better choice than running for someone with severely arthritic knees. Not everyone can squat through a full range of motion or bench with a bar due to shoulder, hip, or knee pain. Not everyone can do high-impact movements. That's okay, there are so many ways to work around these issues and still effectively improve strength, endurance, and cardiovascular conditioning that, barring extreme disability, very few limits exist.

---

54 Mayo Clinic, "Managing Arthritis Pain"; Holger Cramer et al., "Postural Awareness and Its Relation to Pain: Validation of an Innovative Instrument Measuring Awareness of Body Posture in Patients with Chronic Pain," *BMC Musculoskeletal Disorders* 19, no. 1, article no. 109 (April 6, 2018): 9.

55 Alexandro Andrade et al., "A Systematic Review of the Effects of Strength Training in Patients with Fibromyalgia: Clinical Outcomes and Design Considerations," *Advances in Rheumatology* 58, no. 1, article no. 36 (October 22, 2018): 12.; Angela J. Busch et al., "Exercise for Fibromyalgia: A Systematic Review," *The Journal of Rheumatology* 35, no. 6, article no. 1130 (June 1, 2008): 1141–2.

Pain at rest or while moving that isn't linked to a diagnosed injury can be caused by any number of factors. In my experience training clients and myself, many of these pains are simply caused by deficiencies in strength and flexibility (these two attributes are often intrinsically linked) or incorrect movement patterns and posture that developed due to pain or weakness in another part of the body.

Strengthening your joints through a full range of motion not only improves strength, but it also improves flexibility and balance and helps correct poor movement patterns. We all get into bad habits from time to time, and it's worth the effort to correct them. Problems that you do not resolve or get worse over time may require the work of a bodywork specialist such as a massage therapist or chiropractor.

HOW IS YOUR POSTURE AT REST? SITTING? STANDING?

Do you remember being told to sit up straight and not slouch when you were a kid? I remember seeing TV shows and movies depicting women in the fifties learning to drink tea delicately and walk around with books on their heads. My mother used to go after me for leaning on the dinner table, and teachers were always going after us for slouching in our chairs during class. I don't really see this much anymore.

One of the first things I look at when a person comes into my gym for the first time is how they stand and walk. Posture can tell me a lot about a person's strengths and weaknesses. When a person is standing up straight, I want to see that their ear is in line with their shoulder, their shoulders are centered over their hips, and their hips are centered over their midfoot.

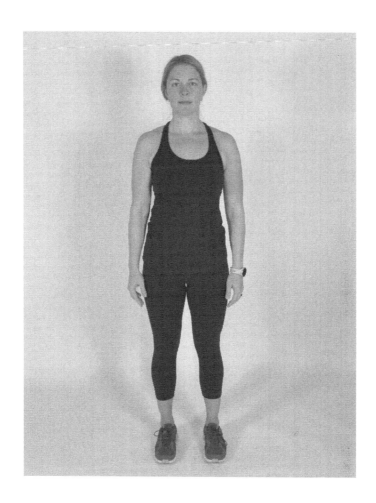

Figure 3.1: Front posture

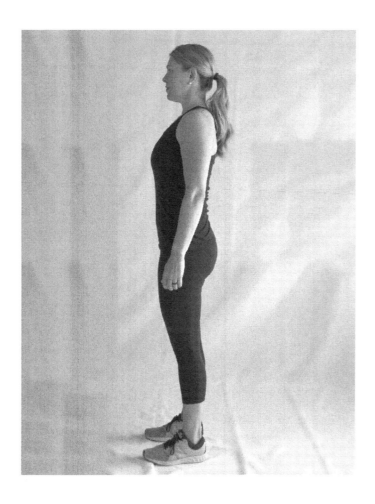

Figure 3.2: Side posture

Where posture breaks down, there is usually a weakness or a lack of flexibility. For example, your typical office worker who sits at a desk all day will typically have rounded shoulders and forward head posture both from a weak upper back and tight hip flexors.

Postural strength, for all intents and purposes, is the ability to maintain one's posture over time or through a series of complex movements. When we can no longer actively support our joints due to weakness or fatigue, we begin to slouch and our posture changes over time. We also lose our balance more easily and become less coordinated. Think about how you feel after a long day at work. If you have a hard time maintaining your posture when you're tired, you lack postural strength.[56]

1. Do you think you have good posture?
2. Can you maintain it all day?
3. Do you find yourself slouching at the end of a long day?

Keep these questions in mind going forward. Some of these issues can be corrected simply by being aware enough to practice good posture regularly. Others will require some dedicated strength and flexibility training. We will discuss this topic more in depth in Chapter Five.

HOW STRONG ARE YOU?

You may have gathered from the last question that strength has a lot to do with posture. Strength begins in our core, i.e., the muscles that support the spine. These tissues include what we think of as abs but are actually all the muscles that surround our torso and abdomen, back and front. When these

---

56 Francesco Carini et al., "Posture and Posturology, Anatomical and Physiological Profiles: Overview and Current State of Art," *Acta Bio-Medica : Atenei Parmensis* 88, no. 1 (April 28, 2017): 11–15.; DeokJu Kim et al., "Effect of an Exercise Program for Posture Correction on Musculoskeletal Pain," *Journal of Physical Therapy Science* 27, no. 6 (June 2015): 1791–94.

muscles are strong, it is easier to control the rest of our body without excessive effort. Our hips are the next important group of muscles, and they are the primary drivers of most power movements such as throwing, sprinting, and jumping. Our upper back and shoulders are equally important in full body movements, and strength in these areas contributes to easy movement, good balance, and power.

Although this may all sound very complicated, I have a very simple test for full body strength, and it is simply this:

How easy is it for you to get up out of a chair?

- Can you simply stand up?
- Do you need to lean forward?
- Do you have to push yourself up with your arms?
- Does it require that you rock back and forth a few times?
- Do you need help?

Your hip and core strength will dictate how easy this task is for you. If you can get up no problem, great! The postural questions above will fill in the rest for us. If you have trouble, we have some work to do.

Don't worry, this problem is actually more easily corrected than you may think.

HOW IS YOUR AEROBIC CONDITIONING?

Our aerobic conditioning can be tested in a great deal of arbitrary ways. Some of the limitations we may have with being able to walk more than a mile may have more to do with endurance and strength than our aerobic capacity. However, since walking is our primary mode of movement, we will answer this question relative to walking. This question is primarily about how easily you get out of breath.

- Do you get out of breath walking up a flight of stairs?
- Walking across the room?
- If you are walking with other people can you carry on a conversation without getting out of breath?
- How far can you comfortably walk without slowing down or needing a break?

WHAT ARE THE FITNESS ROUTINES OR SPORTS YOU HAVE USED IN THE PAST?

We all retain some motor memory of the **fitness routines and sports** we have participated in over the course of our lives. This neurological ability to retain skills after long bouts of not practicing said skill are what we mean when we say, "It's like riding a bike." Research has also shown that changes to our muscles from these activities at the genetic level allow them to rapidly regain strength and size previously developed after long periods of inactivity. To put it simply, you not only retain the long-term skill, but you also retain the ability to rapidly return to the size and strength that enabled that skill.[57]

---

57 Robert A Seaborne et al., "Human Skeletal Muscle Possesses an Epigenetic Memory of Hypertrophy," *Scientific Reports* 8, no. 1, article no. 1898 (January 30, 2018): 12–15.

HOW MUCH TIME PER DAY OR WEEK DO YOU HAVE TO BE ACTIVE?

An underestimated factor in your training plan is simply **how much time you have**. Unless you are a professional athlete, you probably don't have a lot of spare time to spend in the gym. For us everyday folks, work, family, and friends can dominate most of our waking hours. While these commitments are important to living a healthy and happy life, so is exercise. Fitness isn't just for fun, it is for health, quality of life, and, for many of us, much-needed stress relief.

Ideally, thirty minutes a day of physical activity should be enough to decrease most health risks. Instead of thinking of this exercise slot as a single block of time spent in the gym, think about ways you can combine it with your other obligations when necessary. Going for a walk with your family, participating in a recreational league sport, and doing house or yard work are all acceptable ways to be active. If necessary, you can break this hour up into smaller segments throughout your day; ten to fifteen minutes here and there are better than nothing.

You will see in the next few chapters that a big part of improving our health and overall fitness is simply practicing better posture and movement throughout our day. When we become too focused on gym-based workouts being the only path to fitness, we overlook these simpler and more accessible ways to improve our lives.

ARE YOU GOING TO BE TRAINING IN A GYM? AT HOME? WHAT EQUIPMENT IS AVAILABLE TO YOU?

- Where are you going to train?
- What equipment do you have available to you?

A fully equipped gym is not necessary for you to live a fit life. You can work out in your own home, yard, or local park, for example. When we consider the amount of physical activity that is part of your regular day, you may be pleasantly surprised that you don't have to add much more.

HOW IS YOUR BODY COMPOSITION?

Let's be honest, body composition matters to a lot of people, but making body composition change a primary goal is not always the best course of action. As you will see in Chapter Nine, outcome-based goals and extrinsic motivation factors (like appearance) can be counter-productive. However, it is, like everything else here, a data point we should keep track of, especially since it can be related to some health risks.

Measuring body composition can be a sensitive subject and tends to be subjective for a good deal of people, so I am going to keep this relatively simple. Although it is much maligned, BMI (Body Mass Index) is still a relatively good measure of where you lie on the scale of underweight to overweight and obese. People with more muscle will typically have a higher BMI, so we will couple that with two other measures: a waist circumference and scale weight. It is generally accepted that a waist circumference larger than thirty-five inches in women and forty inches in men puts you at a higher risk for cardiovascular disease and diabetes.[58] Some people don't like to weigh themselves; others will obsessively weigh themselves multiple times a day. Understand that your weight can fluctuate up to five or six pounds per day depending on food, sleep, and water intake so take it all with a grain of salt.[59]

Personally, when I have a body composition or weight goal, I weigh myself every morning when I wake up and track it over time, so I know if I need to lower my calories and/or increase my activity levels. Additionally, I take photos of myself in a bikini on a weekly basis, so I can tell if I'm making progress even if the scale isn't showing it. When I'm not cutting weight, I tend to use the old "do my pants still fit?" test. So, pick your test, record your numbers (or photos), and check in regularly.

If you need to gain or lose weight, the most important step is going to be to start tracking your diet. Many of us make assumptions about how much we are eating and drinking, and the truth is, we often greatly underestimate how much that is. Tracking apps such as My Fitness Pal can be a great tool for assessing just how many calories you are taking in every day, in addition to protein, fat, and carbohydrates. In Appendix B, I specifically address why diet plays such an important role in your body composition. Exercise helps; however, a good diet is more important.

* * *

---

58   National Heart, Lung, and Blood Institute, "Assessing Your Weight and Health Risk," US Department of Health and Human Services.

59   Natalie Silver, "Why Does My Weight Fluctuate?" *Healthline*, July 31, 2018.

The most important thing to remember about assessment is that it is ongoing. Regular observation and review of our training log allows us to tell if we are making progress, need an exercise modification, or need a modification to our training plans. In the next few chapters, we will start to learn about some exercises we can use to build our individual fitness routine. Simply recording what exercises we do on a given day will give us a timeline that we can go back to and review to see what progress we've made over time. You will see yourself exercising better, longer, more often, and with more resistance over time.

CHAPTER 4

LET'S GO FOR A WALK

———

Walking has always been a big part of my life. I grew up in the country, where kids pretty much wandered free every waking moment that wasn't required for chores or school. My grandfather had been a game warden, and my father was a science teacher, so I spent countless hours walking in woods and fields with both of them, especially during the fall and winter.

My mother would regularly send my dad and me into the woods and, more importantly, out of her house for errands with requests like, "Gather greenery for Christmas decorations," or, "Bring me that wildflower I saw in the back field," whenever she wanted some alone time. Having a wood burning stove meant lots of scouting trips for downed trees that we would cut up to bring back home to heat the house all winter. It wasn't always work, my best friend and I traveled far distances to terrorize the local frog population (catch and release only) and fall into dark, muddy water whenever possible.

I still love to walk, especially in the woods, and I will walk pretty much anywhere. It's a great way to explore a city, a small town, or enjoy a local park. Lately, I have been spending a lot of time walking not just for my physical health, but also for my mental health.

When COVID-19 first hit the US in early 2020, I had just finished competing at the Lightweight Highland Games National Championships. It was a tough competition, and I had cut close to twenty pounds to make weight (it was right after Christmas, and I am fond of pie). I had trained hard for six weeks to prepare myself for the competition, so my joints and I were understandably ready for a break when it was all over. Unfortunately, this coincided with the sudden and unexpected death of my mother. She and my dad lived right up the street from my family, and she was a welcome part of our daily lives. We were all simply devastated, and then we went into COVID quarantine.

Quite frankly, I did not know what to do with myself. Grief is a funny thing. It's not some cut-and-dry moment of deep sadness—it is confusion, rage, and constant second-guessing about both the past and the future. I couldn't get away from my thoughts, I wasn't sleeping, and I was exhausted all the time. I didn't want to talk to anyone about it because that just opened a big raw wound that I wasn't ready to expose. So, I started getting up with my dog in the very early morning hours and going for walks.

For those first three months of lockdown, I never stepped foot in my basement gym. Instead, I mostly walked. Any time I felt like the darkness was taking over, I put my dog in my car, drove to the woods, and walked for miles. Sometimes I just listened to the early morning chatter of the birds, other times I listened to podcasts and audiobooks. Walking helped me think more clearly, solve problems, and reconnect with myself. When it comes to physical fitness, walking can seem to some to be a rather mediocre way of improving your body, but if you really understand what walking can do for both your body and mind, you will see this amazing activity in a whole new light.

WALKING AND YOUR BRAIN

Walking is the movement our bodies evolved to perform as we developed two-legged locomotion. Our muscles, our bone structure, and our movement patterns are all primarily based on our ability to do that one task. It doesn't stop with just our muscles and bones. Our brains and our organs all function better when we are upright and moving. Walking is extraordinarily and fundamentally essential for our general mobility, our health, our organ function, our cognitive function, and our overall ability to be fully functional human beings.[60]

In his book *In Praise of Walking*, neuroscientist Shane O'Mara takes us on a tour of the brain and explains the intricate role that walking plays in both our general health and in the function of our brain and nervous system. O'Mara's work focuses primarily on cognition, memory, and learning as well as the brain systems affected by stress and depression, and in his book, O'Mara takes a special interest in the brain's

---

60 Shane O'Mara, *In Praise of Walking: The New Science of How We Walk and Why It's Good for Us*, New York: W. W. Norton & Company, 2020: 10–11.

connection to movement. *In Praise of Walking* shows the reader how walking is *the* fundamental primary activity we evolved to perform. In fact, one could make the argument, and he does, that movement is the only thing that required us to have a brain in the first place.[61]

Simply getting up and walking across the room increases blood flow to the brain. Research has shown that even short bouts of low-intensity movement can stimulate the memory and cognitive centers of the brain.[62] Regular walking has been shown to reduce and reverse aging in the brain by stimulating the development of new brain cells in the hippocampus, the learning and memory center of the brain.[63] In fact, regular exercise in the form of walking can actually increase the size of the hippocampus and improve memory in older adults.[64] It plays a role in the treatment of conditions such as Alzheimer's, Parkinson's, decreased cognitive function, and depression and significantly increases cognitive function and development.[65] Just 10 minutes of walking prior to perform-

61   Ibid., 29–30.

62   Kazuya Suwabe et al., "Rapid Stimulation of Human Dentate Gyrus Function with Acute Mild Exercise," *Proceedings of the National Academy of Sciences* 115, no. 41 (October 9, 2018): 10489–90.

63   O'Mara, *In Praise of Walking: The New Science of How We Walk and Why It's Good for Us:* 10–12.

64   Kirk I. Erickson et al., "Exercise Training Increases Size of Hippocampus and Improves Memory," *Proceedings of the National Academy of Sciences* 108, no. 7 (February 15, 2011): 3017–21.

65   Andrea Camaz Deslandes, "Exercise and Mental Health: What Did We Learn in the Last 20 Years?" *Frontiers in Psychiatry* 5 (2014): 66.; Anya Doherty and Anna Forés Miravalles, "Physical Activity and Cognition: Inseparable in the Classroom," *Frontiers in Education* 4:105 (2019): 1–5.

ing a test has been shown to increase high school students' performance in math and memory problems.[66]

Research by anthropologist David Raichlen and psychologist Gene Alexander has shown a relationship between the brain and aerobic physical activity in multiple species. In humans, it is thought that our evolution as endurance-based hunter-gatherers had a direct effect on our brain size and cognitive function. This is based on the observation that brain size increased dramatically in parallel with dramatic increases in our activity level.[67]

Think about it this way, foraging and hunting require a great deal of mental engagement with the environment—planning, mapping, and the ability to travel long distances. In short, the demands of our hunter-gatherer lifestyle gifted us with big brains and a high work capacity. *In order for our bodies and brains to function optimally (and not atrophy), we need regular physical activity that is mentally stimulating.*[68]

66　Erin K. Howie, Jeffrey Schatz, and Russell R. Pate, "Acute Effects of Classroom Exercise Breaks on Executive Function and Math Performance: A Dose-Response Study," *Research Quarterly for Exercise and Sport* 86, no. 3 (2015): 217–218.

67　David A. Raichlen and John D. Polk, "Linking Brains and Brawn: Exercise and the Evolution of Human Neurobiology," *Proceedings of the Royal Society B: Biological Sciences* 280, no. 1750 (January 7, 2013): 6–7.

68　David A. Raichlen and Gene E. Alexander, "Adaptive Capacity: An Evolutionary-Neuroscience Model Linking Exercise, Cognition, and Brain Health," *Trends in Neurosciences* 40, no. 7 (July 2017): 414–5, 418–9.

WE EVOLVED TO NEED PHYSICAL ACTIVITY FOR A HEALTHY BODY AND BRAIN

Herman Pontzer, an evolutionary anthropologist at Duke University, researches how the health and physiology of the human body has evolved. A good portion of his research has been on hunter-gatherers and subsistence farmers in both Africa and South America and how they compare to modern day Westerners in lifestyle, health, and energy expenditure. He has lived among some of these groups and observed their daily activities. Pontzer is known for his studies on human and primate metabolism and has made some rather surprising conclusions about exercise and human health.

In a review article titled "Hunter-gatherers as Models of Public Health," Pontzer and his colleagues refute a few of the more broadly accepted assumptions made popular by the Paleo diet and lifestyle movement that became popular in the early 2000s. It is true that modern day hunter-gatherer and subsistence farmer societies are in much better health overall than Western populations regarding cardiovascular disease, high blood pressure, diabetes, and obesity. Unsurprisingly, the daily activity levels of these populations are much greater than those in Western cultures.[69]

However, the main conclusion of this article, based on countless studies, is that *the daily energy expenditure of modern day hunter-gatherers is the same as that of modern day industrialized populations regardless of activity*

---

69   H. Pontzer, B. M. Wood, and D. A. Raichlen, "Hunter-Gatherers as Models in Public Health," *Obesity Reviews* 19, no. S1 (December 1, 2018): 24–30.

level.[70] Many factors account for this finding, which I explain in more detail in Appendix B: Evolution and Why Diet Is Important, but the main point is that exercise plays a far greater role in our health than it does in weight loss.

As stated in Chapter One, the paradox of our modern lives is that we evolved to conserve energy whenever possible because the physical activity demands of the hunter-gatherer lifestyle were high. Our bodies evolved to reward that physical activity with better brain function and less disease. Our health problems as a species began when foraging and hunting were no longer a part of our modern lives. The physical activity we used to rely on for both food *and good health* is no longer a necessity.

Unlike the modern garage gym fantasy that cavemen engaged in all-day bouts of vigorous sprinting, jumping, climbing, and fighting that has resulted in all kinds of high-intensity, hard and heavy, boot camp-style workouts, modern hunter-gatherers mostly walk. Other activities include digging for tubers, foraging for berries and firewood, carrying water, wood, children, and food, sometimes dancing, and usually a bit of play, especially among the kids who start foraging for themselves as soon as they are old enough not to be carried around by Mom.[71]

Physical activity does not occur in intense short bursts; rather, it tends to consist of moderate sustained activity throughout

---

70 Ibid., 30–34.

71 Vicky Hallett, "Staying Fit Isn't A New Year's Resolution for These Hunter-Gatherers," NPR.org.

the day coupled with plenty of rest. We know this because a team of researchers has been studying the daily activity and health of modern day hunter-gatherers for the past several years. One group, the Hazda in West Africa, were not only observed, but they agreed to wear activity trackers and have blood samples drawn over a two-week period to measure exactly what their days consisted of and how it affected certain physiological markers.[72]

According to the team's observations, the Hazda typically spend about 85–115 minutes per day doing moderate to vigorous physical activities as described above. They, like us, also spend a great deal of time, up to ten hours a day, being non-ambulatory, i.e., not moving. One might assume that it is the 85–115 minutes of moderate to vigorous activity alone that accounts for their overall better health, but is there more to the story?[73]

One research group thinks that there is. In a paper published by Raichlen, et al. in January 2020, the study found that the bigger difference between the Hazda's lifestyle and ours is how we spend our non-ambulatory time. Non-ambulatory activities in hunter-gatherer society are usually spent in what we call "active postures." This means standing, kneeling, or squatting, all three of which stimulate far more muscle activity than the Western tendency to sit or recline in a chair which stimulates virtually no muscle activity at all. Additionally, the duration of these non-ambulatory bouts in

---

72 David A. Raichlen et al., "Sitting, Squatting, and the Evolutionary Biology of Human Inactivity," *Proceedings of the National Academy of Sciences* 117, no. 13 (March 31, 2020): 7119–21.

73 Raichlen et al.: 7117

hunter-gatherers are short, i.e., no more than fifteen minutes on average. In other words, ***they are getting up and moving or changing position multiple times in an hour.***[74]

It may not be our lack of vigorous physical activity that is killing us, it is the predominance of complete inactivity in our schedules that may be the real culprit in our development of disease. Passive sitting and reclining, as we tend to do in most office jobs and leisure time, results in little to no stimulation of muscle activity. I would argue that passive posture in general fails to stimulate a great deal of potential muscle activity in most of our daily activities whether we are resting or not. Look around you—very few people carry themselves with active upright posture whether they are walking, sitting, or standing.

Unfortunately, we already know the catastrophic health results of full body passive rest. Complete inactivity is a known problem in hospitals and care centers where patients are confined to bed rest for any number of reasons. Prolonged bed rest negatively affects multiple organ systems and can even cause new disease and dysfunction regardless of diet or body weight. Muscle weakness, lack of balance, sarcopenia, blood clots, constipation, loss of bone density, glucose

---

74   Ibid. 7115–19.

intolerance, insulin resistance, and high cholesterol are all induced by bed rest, as is anxiety, depression, and insomnia.[75]

Bed rest has similar effects to that which astronauts experience in the zero-gravity environment of space.[76] It's not just the lack of movement, it comes down to not actively resisting gravity. We did not evolve to have inactive muscles, and it has been shown undeniably that our bodies break down very quickly when we are passive in our posture and our movements.

To be like modern day hunter-gatherers and mitigate most health risks, we need to be physically active for two hours a day. More importantly, *we need to resist the urge to sit or move passively when we aren't actively moving.* That doesn't mean running marathons and spending half the day in the gym, it's just moving throughout our day and practicing good posture whenever possible.

If you find yourself sitting in a chair for most of the day due to work, school, or other obligations, make a point to sit with active posture rather than reclining or slouching. Get up a few times every hour and walk around a bit or even just stand up, take a deep breath, lift up your chest, and stretch. If we

75 Luana Petruccio Cabral Monteiro Guedes, Maria Liz Cunha de Oliveira, and Gustavo de Azevedo Carvalho, "Deleterious Effects of Prolonged Bed Rest on the Body Systems of the Elderly—a Review," *Revista Brasileira de Geriatria e Gerontologia* 21 (2018): 500–504.; N. T. Contributor, "Effects of Bedrest 3: Gastrointestinal, Endocrine and Nervous Systems," *Nursing Times* (blog), January 21, 2019.

76 Alan R. Hargens and Laurence Vico, "Long-Duration Bed Rest as an Analog to Microgravity," *Journal of Applied Physiology* 120, no. 8 (February 18, 2016): 891–2.

don't have time to go for a long walk, even a short walk will do. Every little bit helps.

If your job requires that you be on your feet most of the day, guess what? You're likely already getting the physical activity you need. Laborers, health care workers, and postal workers in general get plenty of daily physical activity and unsurprisingly, office workers get the least.[77]

In essence, we were doing just fine as a species until we went and screwed it all up by inventing chairs. Being the clever humans we are, we mechanized a great deal of the work and maintenance usually required for daily life, and we developed jobs that mostly require sitting at a desk. Of course, there is also the television. Sitting in chairs has thrown the proverbial monkey wrench into our evolutionary path to good health.

Yet, there *is* hope.

As stated in Chapter One, the amount of physical activity necessary to restore and maintain good health is not insurmountable. More importantly, it is the avoidance of complete inactivity that is better for our health and mental well-being in the long run. Getting up out of our chairs on a regular basis and going for a walk is truly the best medicine.

---

77 Stephanie A. Prince et al., "Device-Measured Physical Activity, Sedentary Behaviour and Cardiometabolic Health and Fitness across Occupational Groups: A Systematic Review and Meta-Analysis," *The International Journal of Behavioral Nutrition and Physical Activity* 16: 30 (April 2, 2019): 9–11.

IS THERE A RIGHT WAY TO WALK?

Yes, there is.

When you do get an opportunity to walk for exercise, make the most of it. Although walking is one of the most intuitive activities we can engage in, it pays to be self-aware so as to not get into and reinforce bad habits. The most important habit to remember is your posture.

Standing and walking with good posture can strengthen the entire body. Keep your shoulders back and chest up with your head in line with your shoulders. Pull your belly button in toward your spine (this neutralizes excessive curving of the lower spine which can cause lower back pain) and swing your arms with each step. Keep an energetic pace. Don't be passive!

If you have a hard time maintaining good posture while walking, it's okay, many people do at first. It will get better with practice and the next couple of chapters on strength training can help with improving your form as well. If you recall from Chapter Two, the most important part of training whether you are training for the Olympics or just getting back to an active lifestyle is *accumulating a higher volume of good quality work.*

RUCKING

Some folks feel that walking alone is not enough of a fitness challenge, and this may be true for the more fit among us. For this reason, rucking, or walking with a weighted vest or pack, has become more popular in recent years. Rucking with weight can increase the cardiovascular stress of regular walking as well as build strength in the upper back, core, and legs. A lot of us, especially kids with their school backpacks, are already doing this without even realizing it.

Rucking with a backpack can sometimes lead to shoulder and neck pain from the compression of the straps and the forward head position some people adopt to maintain their balance. If this occurs, it is important that you reduce the weight of your pack and be mindful that your posture is in the correct position. Wearing a hip belt and taking more frequent breaks can help as well.[78] Some people new to rucking may also experience foot and ankle pain. To avoid these injuries, be cognizant that your shoes are just as important as your rucking equipment.

Start with relatively light weights, perhaps between five to ten pounds, and increase weights conservatively, i.e., approximately five pounds per week. You will want to be conservative with your frequency and distance. Most beginners should start off with one to two miles, two to three times per week.[79]

Many online resources exist for both rucking equipment and programming as well as rucking events. I highly recommend you check some out if you are considering making rucking part of your routine. Rucking.com and RuckforMiles.com are both good places to start.

---

78   "Ruck March Shoulder Pain," How to Avoid It | Ruck for Miles.

79   "Training Program for New Ruckers," *Rucking.Com* (blog), November 10, 2018.

TREKKING AND NORDIC WALKING

A few years back, I wrote a group training certification course for the International Sports Sciences Association that encouraged students to come up with their own creative group fitness classes. One of my students designed her class around the concept of Nordic walking.

You've probably seen people on hiking trails holding on to a set of poles that they use to help propel themselves forward. I used to think that these were simply a tool for those who were not steady on their feet or needed a little help to move more efficiently. This is not an incorrect assumption; they are well suited for that purpose. However, these poles are also very powerful tools for turning ordinary walking into a much more effective full body workout. Actively pushing off the poles while walking engages more muscles than walking alone, especially those in the upper back, shoulder, and arms. This method reduces stress on the lower extremities, which makes it easier on those who suffer chronic back, hip, and knee pain.

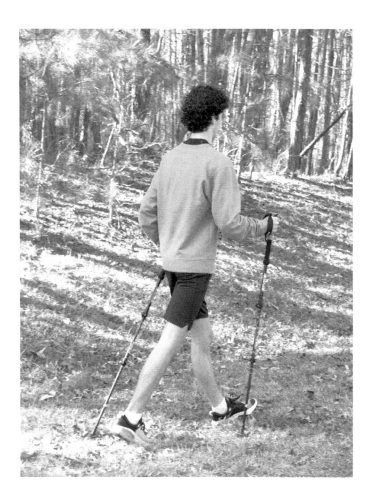

Figure 4.1: Photo of Nordic Walking

My student, a very fit woman in her late sixties, had designed a class where she gathered individuals at a local park and took them on fast-paced Nordic walks around it. She stopped at regular intervals during the walk where the less fit individuals could rest while the more fit individuals would perform some bodyweight exercises such as squats and push-ups. It turned out to be a very popular class with a mixture of both old and young participants. Whether you need the extra stability provided by the poles or simply want a more full-body workout from your daily walks, Nordic walking is a great option regardless of your age and fitness level, and the stability the poles provide makes walking on uneven terrain, like unpaved paths and trails, more feasible for those who would otherwise avoid it.

As stated above, many people tend to use walking poles simply for added stability, and in this capacity, they are often referred to simply as trekking poles. However, to properly Nordic walk, there is an actual technique to using them that makes them very effective for increasing speed and stability. Increasing speed is the primary goal of Nordic walking, and, as I mentioned above, gait speed is another variable that relates to cognitive decline. Again, there are many online resources, including equipment and technique videos, that can help you incorporate Nordic walking into your routine.[80]

The Nordic walking technique is a simple enhancement of normal arm swing when walking. The poles remain behind the body and point diagonally backward at all times.

- *Shoulders are relaxed and down.*
- *Poles are held close to the body.*
- *The hands are opened slightly to allow the poles to swing forward—the poles are not gripped, rather they swing from the wrist straps.*

---

80 "Add Confidence and Stability on the Trails with Trekking Poles," Verywell Fit.

- *The leading foot strikes the ground.*
- *The opposite arm swings forward to waist height.*
- *The opposite pole strikes the ground level with the heel of the opposite foot.*
- *The poles remain pointing diagonally backward, they are never in front of the body.*
- *Push the pole as far back as possible, the arm straightening to form a continuous line with the fully extended arm, the hand opening off the grip by the end of the arm swing.*
- *The foot rolls through the step to push off with the toe. This lengthens the stride behind the body, getting the most out of each stride.*
- *The arm motion is loose and relaxed.*

Keeping the arms relaxed and keeping the poles behind the body are key elements in the proper technique. Many people use the wrong technique, planting the poles in front of the body and bending the elbow too much.[81]

A good online resource for Nordic walking is americannordicwalking.com.

EVERYTHING ELSE

Walking and virtually anything you can do to move your body over a sustained period is going to help improve your health and cognition. Weight-bearing exercises such as walking, running, dancing, or playing tennis are all going to benefit your general health **and** your bone health. Non-weight bearing activities such as rowing, cycling, or swimming are

---

81   "What Is Nordic Walking?" Verywell Fit.

still advantageous, but some sort of weight-bearing exercise such as walking or lifting weights is needed to maintain bone density.[82] For overweight individuals, getting into the water can provide an opportunity to move while decreasing pressure on their spine and joints. In general, any kind of movement is going to stimulate our brains and bodies for the better.

The take-home message here is that whether you walk unloaded, walk with weight, use a walking stick or poles, run, dance, bike, or swim, moving with good posture and purpose not only keeps your body healthy, but it also keeps your mind healthy as well. These benefits are not as obvious during our youth. The older folks around us tell a different story. If you pay attention, you will see that *those who move well are those who think and live well.*

ASSESSING YOUR DAILY ACTIVITY

For good health, the CDC recommends a minimum of five thousand steps per day. That's the equivalence of about 2.2 miles.[83] If you aren't sure how many steps you are taking daily, pedometers and activity trackers are great ways to assess that. It is this daily assessment that allows us to see exactly how much exercise we are getting. If we aren't getting

---

82   "Exercise for Your Bone Health," NIH Osteoporosis and Related Bone Diseases National Resource Center.

83   Adrienne Santos-Longhurst, "Average Steps Per Day by Age, Gender, Occupation, and Country."

enough, then we know that we need to modify our behavior to get in more steps when we can and need to.[84]

If you don't already engage in regular cardiovascular exercise, start by assessing how many hours you sit, stand, or move throughout the day. If you have an active job, you may already be getting your daily requirement of movement; however, if your job is largely sedentary, assess how often you get up and walk around. A very easy trick for remembering to get up and move more regularly is to increase your water intake. Drinking a half to a full gallon of water a day is not only good for you, it will also ensure that you have to make regular trips to the bathroom.

For better health, engaging in sustained exercise is more ideal than taking short trips to the restroom and intermittently standing. A more ambitious goal of ten to fifteen thousand steps per day is even more ideal for health and overall fitness. As a mother of three kids with a busy schedule myself, I know it's not always easy to set aside time for devoted exercise, so as we discussed in Chapter Three, it is perfectly okay to break up your exercise into ten- to fifteen-minute chunks. Some of you may be meeting that threshold by walking to and from work or your local shops, which is another great reason to employ the use of a pedometer or activity tracker. If not, could you walk around the parking lot, a nearby mall, or a local park for twenty minutes on your lunch break?

---

84 Alycia N. Sullivan and Margie E. Lachman, "Behavior Change with Fitness Technology in Sedentary Adults: A Review of the Evidence for Increasing Physical Activity," *Frontiers in Public Health* 4: 289 (January 11, 2017).

If you are already engaging in regular cardiovascular exercise, keep track of what you do, when you do it, and how long (time or distance) you do it for. How many miles a week are you running/walking/rowing, etc.? If you aren't training for anything in particular, think about how much time you are devoting to that exercise. If you're meeting your weekly requirement of two-and-a-half to five hours or more, we can start thinking about replacing some of that time with improving your overall fitness by building some strength.

Sustained activity at a moderate pace for thirty to forty-five minutes, three to five times per week is the traditional way we think about getting our cardiovascular exercise, and it is more effective at producing the cardiovascular changes that improve our aerobic fitness. However, if you just aren't there yet, hopefully you can see that any amount of standing, walking, and moving is going to change your health and brain function for the better. The healthier and more fit you become, the more you will be able to do. As you move more, more often, and for longer periods of time, your overall strength and health will improve. When we feel good, we move more without even thinking about it.

* * *

Our bodies evolved to be active, and walking is the most natural physical activity for our bodies to engage in. Walking improves brain function and memory, keeps our bodies healthy, and staves off depression. For optimal functioning of all our organ systems, especially the immune and nervous system, we need to be regularly physically active throughout our day. Inactivity, regardless of body size, is the primary cause in the development of heart disease, diabetes, some cancers, muscle loss, and cognitive decline. If nothing else, if you can get out and walk every day, you will be far healthier than if you don't.

CHAPTER 5

STRENGTH TRAINING: THE ART AND THE TOOLS

While walking is extremely well suited for achieving our daily activity level, we still have to work to ensure that our bodies are in top working order and can keep us moving well to decrease the risk of pain and injury. Shoring up our posture, strengthening joints that may have become weak or unbalanced, and building some muscle mass are all feats easily achieved by adding some strength training to your weekly routine.

Strength training, to me, is an art. The goal of strength training in my gym is to take an individual and figure out how to build them a strong, functional body based on their unique traits and goals. In this chapter, I would like to teach you how to become the artist using exercises as the tools we use to build our bodies into functional, efficient machines. The tools that work for you, the individual, may be different from the tools that work for others.

ADAPTATIONS TO STRENGTH TRAINING

As we discussed in Chapter One, strength training is largely neurological. The first six to twelve weeks of a strength program are going to improve your coordination, endurance, and your ability to exert force. Most of that progress is the result of your nervous system learning how to recruit higher numbers of muscle fibers in more muscles more efficiently. To put it simply, your brain is going to learn how to communicate with your muscles and individual muscle fibers and get them working together better. This is why we need to think of strength training as skill development and practice good form and execution. If we simply go through the motions without focusing on correct technique, we risk wasting our efforts.

Strength training works by having your muscles work against some sort of resistance. Resistance can be any number of things, including the following:

1. Your own bodyweight, as in push-ups, pull-ups, or body-weight squats.
2. Weighted objects such as dumbbells, kettlebells, barbells, medicine balls, sandbags, cinder blocks, small children, etc.
3. Elastic bands attached to a stationary object, pulled between two muscle groups, or held by a partner.

It has been shown that the greater the resistance, the greater the effect of strength training on the nervous system.[85]

We want to use weights that are challenging but still allow us to complete the prescribed number of repetitions with good form. We do not want to train to the point of form breakdown or the inability to finish the workout, so choose your weights wisely.

WHAT KIND OF STRENGTH TRAINING DO OUR BODIES NEED?

In general, the following is true:

*For full body strength, the **major joints** must be strong through a **full range of motion** and in concert with the **muscles that support the spine**.*

So, what exactly does that mean? Let's address each of those points.

When we talk about the **major joints**, I am primarily referring to, from the top down, the shoulders, elbows, hips, and knees. Ankles and wrists are important as well, but most exercises that strengthen the elbows and knees are going to strengthen those joints as well.

The **muscles that support the spine** include what we think of as our "core." These tissues are the muscles of our abdomen and lower back as well as the mid and upper back and the

---

85 Nathaniel D. M. Jenkins et al., "Greater Neural Adaptations Following High- vs. Low-Load Resistance Training," *Frontiers in Physiology* 8:331 (2017): 10–13.

muscles of our hips, i.e., our glutes and hip flexors. There are several ways to approach strengthening these joints, and for beginners, the more efficient approach is to emphasize exercises that target large muscle groups and multiple joints whenever possible.

Full-Range-of-Motion is kind of a loaded term when it comes to strength training, and I like to think of this notion as more of a starting ideal rather than a day-one requirement. Range of motion refers to how far your joints flex and extend through a movement. For some bodies, the ideal range of motion for a particular exercise may be very different from other body types. A simple example of this is the difference in individuals' ability to do the splits. Some people can, some people can't; a number of reasons can affect a person's flexibility.

The first reason is that not everyone has the potential for free range of motion in all their joints. Why? The answer lies within the state of the bony structures and connective tissue within the joint itself. Short of surgery, nothing will change the structure of the joint, so, if necessary, we find a workaround.

An example of this is the acromion process, a bony protrusion on the upper outside edge of the shoulder blade. It has three different ways it can present in individuals that range from flat to a hook shape. This hook-shaped version can result in "shoulder impingement syndrome," and individuals with this shape may develop pain with overhead movements.[86]

To accommodate these folks, we can adjust their grip, limit resistance, or change the angle of the exercise. I happen to have this hook-shaped version, so overhead pressing with a bar tends to cause me pain and has led to injury in the past. I have found that pressing with dumbbells instead, with my palms facing one another (instead of toward the front as I would do with a bar) alleviates any problems I would otherwise have.

The second factor is an individual's anthropometry, or the relative measurements of the body, such as limb length, trunk length, and height, may limit an individual's ability to hit certain positions. For example, individuals with long legs have a harder time squatting to full depth than shorter individuals, and that's perfectly fine. As long as you are squatting in a way that is strengthening the targeted muscles, depth is not all that important.

Finally, many range-of-motion issues are related to the "tightness" of a muscle. We often think this means we need to stretch more; however, that's not the whole story. Although tight muscles can be the result of injury, stress, or even dehydration, a lot of times, they are the result of weakness somewhere else.[87] When we have a "tight" muscle, it isn't that the muscle is too short, it is often that the opposing muscle, the

86   Julie A. Creech and Sabrina Silver, "Shoulder Impingement Syndrome," in *StatPearls* (Treasure Island (FL): StatPearls Publishing, 2020).

87   "What Causes Muscle Rigidity?" Healthline, July 5, 2019.

one that controls the opposite or complementary movement, is weak.[88]

Wait, what?

Our nervous system plays many roles in movement, and one of those roles is to protect us from injury by tightening some muscles to pick up the slack for others that are too weak or inactive to do their job correctly. For example, tight hamstrings are often the result of weak glutes, the muscles of your backside.[89] Tight chest muscles can be a symptom of overworked or weak upper back muscles.[90] A tight and painful lower back can be caused by weak core muscles.[91]

What does that mean?

It means that although stretching can temporarily help loosen tight muscles, full-body strength training that balances complementary muscle groups provides a more long-term effect. This does not mean you shouldn't stretch a tight muscle, especially if it's causing you some pain. However, a combination of strength training and stretching is far more effective for improving flexibility than stretching alone.

---

88 "Tips for Understanding Muscle Imbalances," Dynamic Fitness.

89 Harvard Health Publishing, "Are Your Hamstrings Working Double Duty?" *Harvard Health*.

90 "Upper Crossed Syndrome: Causes, Symptoms, and Exercises," Medical News Today, Published August 11, 2017.

91 Satoshi Kato et al., "Abdominal Trunk Muscle Weakness and Its Association with Chronic Low Back Pain and Risk of Falling in Older Women," *BMC Musculoskeletal Disorders* 20: 273 (June 3, 2019).

IS STRENGTH TRAINING SAFE FOR EVERYONE?

Yes.

More importantly, it is essential.

It has been shown that a lack of strength and muscle mass has a direct correlation to early mortality. Strength training improves bone density in postmenopausal women and can actually reverse chronic back and joint pain. It turns back the clock, revs up our metabolism, prevents injury, reverses some medical conditions such as type 2 diabetes and cardiovascular disease, and gives us freedom of mobility and independence long into our twilight years.[92]

Sarcopenia, which begins in our forties, can cause us to lose up to half of our muscle mass by our seventies while our healthy muscle is replaced with fibrous tissue and fat. Sarcopenia is associated with osteoporosis, poor mobility, and early death. There is no medicine that will treat sarcopenia—regular exercise is the only remedy. Even more effective is resistance training.[93]

---

92 Michael McLeod et al., "Live Strong and Prosper: The Importance of Skeletal Muscle Strength for Healthy Ageing," *Biogerontology* 17, no. 3 (June 2016): 497–506.

93 Ronenn Roubenoff, "Sarcopenia: Effects on Body Composition and Function," *The Journals of Gerontology. Series A, Biological Sciences and Medical Sciences* 58 (December 1, 2003): 1012.

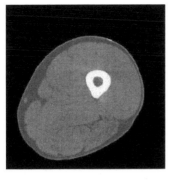 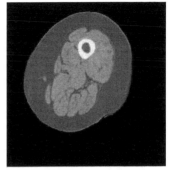

Young, active   Old, sedentary

Figure 5.0: Sarcopenia

In the LIFTMOR study, women in their sixties safely participated in a protocol that included deadlifts, squats, and overhead presses in a strength training format that significantly
improved their bone mineral density.[94] In a review article
of over twenty studies, it was shown that even individuals
over the age of eighty years old can still improve strength
and muscle mass with resistance training. It is never too late
to start getting stronger.[95]

Big, full body movements such as squats, presses, deadlifts,
lunges, etc. contribute to quality of life, longevity, improved

---

94   Steven L. Watson et al., "High-Intensity Resistance and Impact Training
     Improves Bone Mineral Density and Physical Function in Postmeno-
     pausal Women with Osteopenia and Osteoporosis: The LIFTMOR Ran-
     domized Controlled Trial," *Journal of Bone and Mineral Research* 33, no.
     2 (February 1, 2018): 216–219.

95   Jozo Grgic et al., "Effects of Resistance Training on Muscle Size and
     Strength in Very Elderly Adults: A Systematic Review and Meta-Analysis
     of Randomized Controlled Trials," *Sports Medicine* 50, no. 11 (November
     1, 2020): 1983–97.

health, and freedom from pain. Whatever movements you use, if they are appropriately loaded and performed with consistent, good form, you can continue to build strength safely into your twilight years. By strength training, you are building and improving your body the same way a mechanic builds and improves a machine. It really is that simple. For most people, no matter what their daily activities consist of, if you can get stronger, you will live better.

ESSENTIAL FOUNDATIONS OF STRENGTH TRAINING

POSTURE AND CENTER OF GRAVITY

When I first start training someone in my gym, we start by talking about their posture. I tell them what looks good and what they need to pay attention to and work on. As we start learning exercises, I am essentially teaching them how to perform movements with correct posture. Correct posture is incredibly important for joint health and full body function, and it is something we can practice every day simply by being aware of how we are holding ourselves.[96] In fact, a whole industry has been emerging with all kinds of braces and devices designed to remind you to stand up straight, shoulders back, chest up, with ears in line with shoulders.[97]

---

96 Francesco Carini et al., "Posture and Posturology, Anatomical and Physiological Profiles: Overview and Current State of Art," *Acta Bio-Medica : Atenei Parmensis* 88, no. 1 (April 28, 2017): 11–15.

97 Ravi Charan Ailneni et al., "Influence of the Wearable Posture Correction Sensor on Head and Neck Posture: Sitting and Standing Workstations," *Work* 62, no. 1 (2019): 27.

Good upper body posture allows us to breathe more deeply, prevents us from putting unnecessary weight on our necks from forward-leaning heads, and strengthens our upper back. Good posture enables us to move correctly, with good balance. Again, think of those ballroom dancers with their beautiful carriage and seamless movements. *That's what strong looks like.*

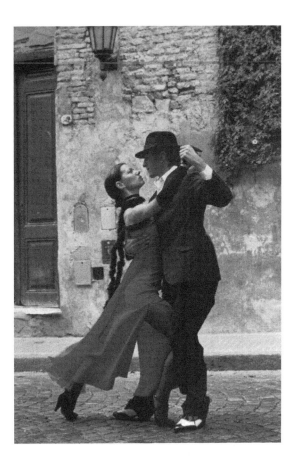

Figure 5.1: Dancers

According to an article in Harvard Health Publishing, good posture can be defined as follows:

- *chin parallel to the floor*
- *shoulders even (roll your shoulders up, back, and down to help achieve this)*
- *neutral spine (no flexing or arching to overemphasize the curve in your lower back)*
- *arms at your sides with elbows straight and even*
- *abdominal muscles braced*
- *hips even*
- *knees even and pointing straight ahead*
- *body weight distributed evenly on both feet*
- *When sitting down, keep your chin parallel to the floor; your shoulders, hips, and knees at even heights; and your knees and feet pointing straight ahead.*[98]

To properly assess your posture, you're going to want to look at yourself from both a front and a side position. Use the cues listed above to be in the best position before making any observations. Use a mirror or camera or even another person to assess your posture as follows:

When observing yourself from the front, you are simply looking for symmetry between the left and right side of the body. Are the left and right sides of your hips and shoulders at the same height? Do you notice any other differences? The truth is, we aren't perfectly symmetrical, so you may see some minor deviations. See if you can adjust your posture to

98 Harvard Health Publishing, "Why Good Posture Matters," *Harvard Health*.

correct anything you see. If you can, then this might simply be a bad habit that you can fix once you are aware of it.

Sometimes these asymmetries can become a bit more permanent and may require some massage, physical therapy, or chiropractic work to correct. Some deviations may be developmental. Scoliosis is a condition that develops in adolescence and causes lateral curvature of the spine (the spine curves sideways.) Some cases of scoliosis are so mild that they aren't noticed and/or don't require treatment, but they can still cause you to stand asymmetrically.[99]

When you turn to your side, you may want to have somebody take a video or a picture of you if you can't do it yourself. Look at figure 5.2. In this photo, Patrick's body is in alignment from the head down to the feet. His head is squarely over his shoulders, with the middle of his ear over his shoulder, and his shoulder is over his hips. His hips are over his midfoot to heel area. If you were to draw a straight line down the length of his body, it should go through the middle of his ear, through his shoulder, through the middle of his hips, and down into his heel or midfoot.

99   "Scoliosis: Treatment, Symptoms, and Causes," Medical News Today, Published March 17, 2020.

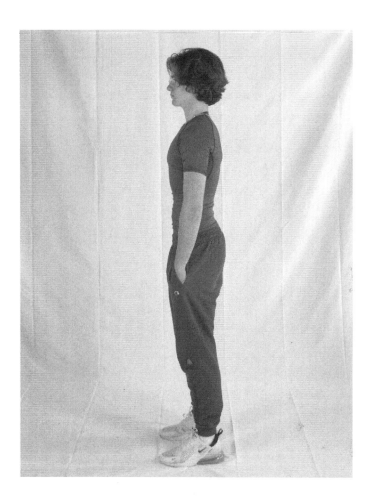

Figure 5.2: Normal Posture

In figure 5.3, Patrick has some excessive inward curvature in his lower back. This is referred to as lordosis, or swayback. We don't want to see any excess rounding of the upper back, or curvature of the lower back. His hips are tilted back, and his abdomen is pushed forward. This position shifts his center of gravity forward to his toes and puts more force on the front side of the vertebrae instead of distributing it evenly. To correct this, he should pull his belly button into his spine and push his hips forward. This will evenly distribute his weight across the full surface of each vertebrae as well as shift his center of gravity back over his midfoot.[100]

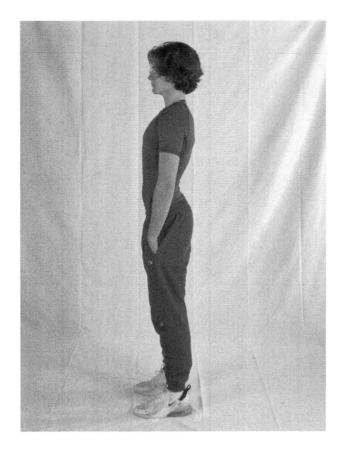

Figure 5.3: Lordosis

100 "Lordosis: Symptoms, Causes, Treatments, and Exercises," Medical News Today, Published June 18, 2020.

In figure 5.4, Patrick is demonstrating rounding of the upper back, or kyphosis. This postural deviation is common in office workers and is becoming more and more common in young people from spending too much time slouched over computers and phones. His shoulders are slumped forward, and his chest is passive, i.e., not open and up. This brings his head posture forward as well as his center of gravity and as a result, he has some excessive lower back curvature to compensate for this. Forward head posture is extremely unfavorable as it can cause remodeling of the spine over time, which, in turn, can cause several other problems such as chronic pain and immobility.[101]

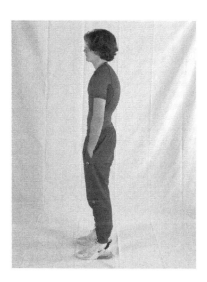

Figure 5.4: Kyphosis

---

101 "Kyphosis: Symptoms, Causes, Exercises, and Treatment," Medical News Today, Published January 2, 2019.; "Rounded Shoulders: Causes, Risk Factors, Diagnosis, and Exercises," Medical News Today, Published July 25, 2017.

Curvature of the lower spine is appropriate when we are specifically training those muscles such as when performing a "Superman" or other back extension. Likewise, rounding of the upper spine can be appropriate when lifting large and/ or awkward objects that require us to wrap our chest and arms around them. However, when performing any other loaded movement, the spine needs to be neutral and relatively straight to prevent injury to both the individual vertebrae and also the cartilage, tendons, ligaments, and nerves that surround them.

In figure 5.5, Francis is performing a "Superman" exercise that requires him to flex his lower back, so his spine curves.

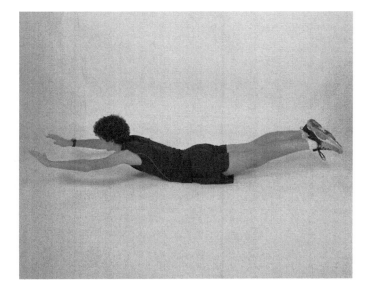

Figure 5.5: Superman

In figure 5.6, Francis is doing a "good morning" exercise to strengthen his hips and stabilize his back, so his spine remains straight.

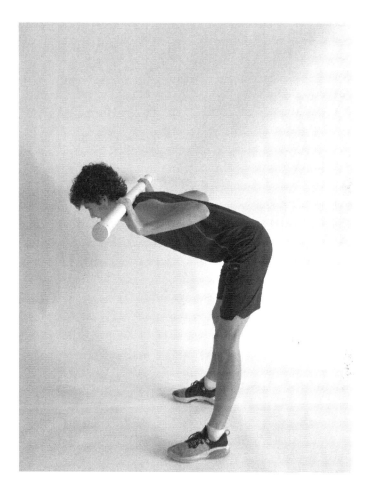

Figure 5.6: Good Morning

Good posture is important because it is the way our bodies evolved to optimally utilize our **center of gravity**. Center of gravity refers to the focal point of gravitational pull on the human body. For most people standing, that is somewhere above or below the navel. Your ability to balance is reliant on where your center of gravity is relative to your base. Your base is your feet. If you were to simply lean to one side as far as you could, eventually, your center of gravity would shift too far away from your base and you would fall.[102]

Center of gravity is important when we pick up a heavy object, and it can be used to our advantage. For example, if you are having trouble getting your hips back on a squat, try holding a weight out in front of you with both hands as in figure 5.7. This shifts your center of gravity forward and therefore allows us to push our hips back farther without falling backward.

102 P. Davidovits, *Physics in Biology and Medicine*, Complementary Science (Elsevier Science, 2012): 2–7.

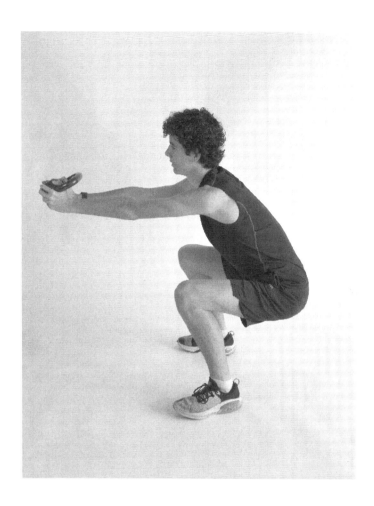

Figure 5.7: Goblet Squat

YOUR CORE

Your core muscles are responsible for stabilizing your core, that big gap you have between your ribcage and your pelvis. They allow you to bend over and stand back up, lean over sideways, and rotate your upper body perpendicular to your hips.

Our core muscles are not just our rectus abdominis, i.e., the muscles in the front that make up the "six-pack"—several muscles make up the musculature all the way around our midsection, including our lower back. These muscles include the obliques, transversus abdominis, erector spinae, and so on.[103]

They are often assisted by the muscle groups that lie directly below and above them, including the glutes, latissimus dorsi, and the hip flexors, such as the rectus femoris and the psoas.[104] It is not necessary that you memorize all these muscles and their actions, it is only necessary that you understand how the core controls stability and movement.

We call it the core because it is the center of your body and consequently, the center of all other movement. When the core muscles are weak, ordinary activities such as getting up out of a chair or rolling over in bed can be unnecessarily taxing. The core muscles give us an abundance of flexibility to rotate and bend while also supporting the spine under load. This ability to stabilize and move in multiple directions

103 Kevin Seeras et al., "Anatomy, Abdomen and Pelvis, Anterolateral Abdominal Wall," in *StatPearls* (Treasure Island (FL): StatPearls Publishing, 2020); Brett Sassack and Jonathan D. Carrier, "Anatomy, Back, Lumbar Spine," in *StatPearls* (Treasure Island (FL): StatPearls Publishing, 2020).

104 Alyssa L. Ransom, Margaret A. Sinkler, and Shivajee V. Nallamothu, "Anatomy, Bony Pelvis and Lower Limb, Femoral Muscles," in *StatPearls* (Treasure Island (FL): StatPearls Publishing, 2020).

allows us to react quickly to regain our balance or change direction when necessary.

Since the core plays such a vital role is postural stability, you can strengthen your core significantly simply by practicing good posture and actively stabilizing those muscles. Movements such as squats, deadlifts, push-ups, and overhead presses all require core stability to perform effectively, and, in turn, significantly strengthen our core muscles. This strengthening occurs during the simple motion of walking, provided you are actively pulling your shoulders back, your chest up, and your belly in.

Stability of our spine is very important, but our core muscles do so much more than that. They allow you to rotate your shoulders independent of your hips and allow you to bend backwards, forwards, and sideways at the waist. Our hips and shoulders both rotate as part of our natural gait cycle, which includes walking or running. The almost infinite combinations of these motions make up some of the most incredible athletic feats we see in gymnastics, wrestling, track and field, basketball, diving, figure skating…the list goes on.

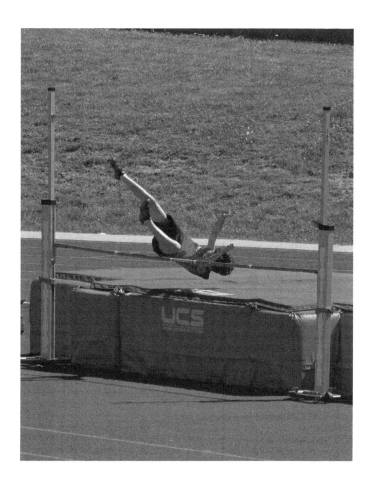

Figure 5.8: High Jump

YOUR HIPS AND LEGS

Moving down from the core, we have the power center of your body: your hips. Your hips consist primarily of the gluteus muscles: the gluteus maximus, gluteus medius, and the gluteus minimus. The gluteus maximus, of course, is the largest muscle that we have, and it is responsible for the shape of our backside. The gluteus maximus is primarily responsible for us being able to stand upright, rise from a sitting position, walk up a hill or stairs, and run.[105]

The gluteus medius, which sits on the side of our gluteus maximus, works to externally rotate the hip and stabilize the pelvis. It performs this function with some assistance from the gluteus minimus, which sits directly under the gluteus maximus. These actions are extremely important because they provide the necessary hip rotation and pelvic stability that is required when walking, running, or doing any movement that requires moving one leg at a time. A lot of knee pain can be tied directly to weakness of the gluteus medius, which prevents the knee from being stable and therefore moving consistently as we walk or run.[106]

The quadriceps are actually a set of four muscles that make up the front of our thigh. They are responsible for bending at the hips, straightening the knee, and like the glutes, they help us maintain our posture and stabilize the knee.[107] The hamstrings are a group of three muscles on the back of the

105 Adel Elzanie and Judith Borger, "Anatomy, Bony Pelvis and Lower Limb, Gluteus Maximus Muscle," in *StatPearls* (Treasure Island (FL): StatPearls Publishing, 2020).

106 TrueSports, "Hip Muscle Weakness Can Cause Knee Pain and Injury," True Sports Physical Therapy, January 22, 2020.

107 Bruno Bordoni and Matthew Varacallo, "Anatomy, Bony Pelvis and Lower Limb, Thigh Quadriceps Muscle," in *StatPearls* (Treasure Island (FL): StatPearls Publishing, 2020).

thigh that are responsible for extending the hip, bending the knee, and stabilizing our posture.[108]

Below the knee, the biggest muscles we see are the gastrocnemius and the soleus of our calf, which join together at the Achilles tendon.[109] These muscles are responsible for flexing and extending our ankle. It should go without saying that all three of these muscle groups, in combination with our hips, are responsible for most of our locomotion, including walking, running, and jumping.

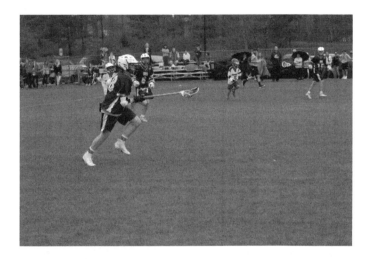

Figure 5.9: Lacrosse Player

108 Jacob E. Vaughn and Wayne B. Cohen-Levy, "Anatomy, Bony Pelvis and Lower Limb, Posterior Thigh Muscles," in *StatPearls* (Treasure Island (FL): StatPearls Publishing, 2020).

109 Justin T. Binstead, Akul Munjal, and Matthew Varacallo, "Anatomy, Bony Pelvis and Lower Limb, Calf," in *StatPearls* (Treasure Island (FL): StatPearls Publishing, 2020).

What is important is that you understand that our legs and hips are an important part of our posture and locomotion. Since we walk on two legs, our legs and hips take on the bulk of the stress of our movement. Strengthening these muscles, as well as the bones and connective tissue that supports ankles, knees, and hips, is incredibly important in maintaining our mobility without injury as we age.

YOUR SHOULDERS AND ARMS

The hips, unlike the shoulders, are relatively stable due to the size and structure of the pelvis. The shoulders, on the other hand, don't have any bony structures providing direct support. Instead, the head of the humerus (the top of the upper arm bone) is largely held in place by the muscles of the rotator cuff and the tendons of the triceps and biceps. This positioning grants more freedom of movement, but it puts a lot of demand on the surrounding muscles and connective tissue in order to stabilize the joint to prevent injury and dislocation.[110]

Aside from the deltoids, those visible muscles that cap the upper arm, at least seventeen other muscles are responsible for stabilizing and moving the shoulder, including muscles of the upper arm, chest, and upper back. As a result, many of the exercises that we will be using for these other muscle groups will have some carryover to shoulder strength and stability.[111]

---

110 Mohammed A. Miniato, Prashanth Anand, and Matthew Varacallo, "Anatomy, Shoulder and Upper Limb, Shoulder," in *StatPearls* (Treasure Island (FL): StatPearls Publishing, 2020).

111 Ibid.

The biceps and triceps are closely involved with stabilizing the shoulder joint, so elbow flexion and extension should be a part of your training program as well. These movements are not just limited to bicep curls and tricep extensions, they are a part of most pressing and pulling movements as well. Pull-ups, push-ups, rows, dips, bench press, and overhead presses all require us to bend our elbows.

Sometimes it's okay to not have any direct arm work in our programs if we have these other movements, however it's always a good idea to include them when we can. The biceps are not only responsible for flexing the elbow, but they are also responsible for rotating the forearm from a palm up to a palm down position, so introducing some rotation into our arm movements is important as well.

YOUR CHEST AND BACK

The muscles of the back are pretty much continuous from the hips to the back of the head. They act in concert with the hips, core, shoulders, and even the arms, so it is hard to separate them as their own entities. The largest muscles of the back, the latissimus dorsi (lats) and the trapezius (traps) are responsible for moving the shoulder blades and the arms to lift and pull in multiple directions. In concert with the many other muscles of the back, they are responsible for stabilizing the spine and maintaining upright posture.[112]

---

112 "Latissimus Dorsi Muscle," Kenhub; Jared Ourieff, Brent Scheckel, and Amit Agarwal, "Anatomy, Back, Trapezius," in *StatPearls* (Treasure Island (FL): StatPearls Publishing, 2020).

The muscles of the chest, the pectoralis major and pectoralis minor, like the muscles of the back, act in concert with the shoulders, arms, and core and complement many of the movements of the upper back. The chest muscles are an important part of the body to pay attention to and are often a problem area related to posture. Tight chest muscles can pull the shoulders forward, resulting in kyphosis, or rounded upper back posture, as shown in figure 5.4. This tightness, however, is often the result of weak upper back muscles, so both stretching the chest muscles and strengthening the upper back is very important for correcting rounded posture.[113]

To stretch these muscles, simply lift your chest and arms and move your arms back until you feel a stretch. Additionally, you can brace your arm in a doorway or against a wall and turn away from your shoulder.

---

113 "Tight Chest Muscles: Why Your Upper Back Is the Key to Their Release," Laguna Orthopedic Rehabilitation.

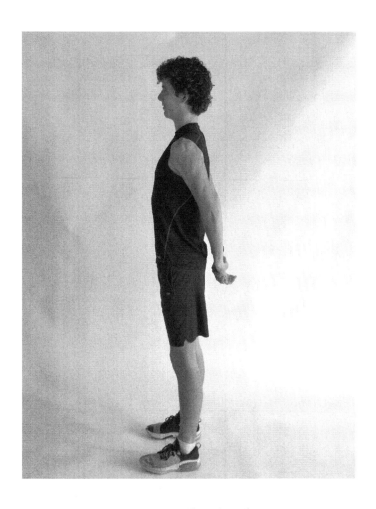

Figure 5.10a: Chest Stretch 1

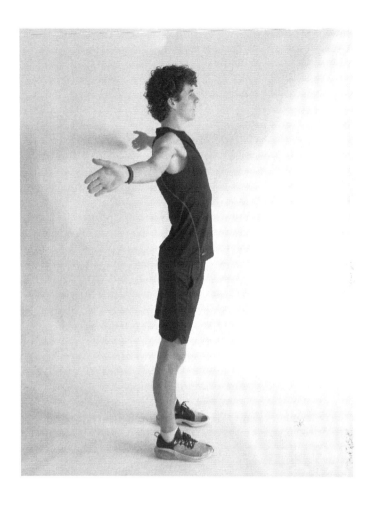

Figure 5.10b: Chest Stretch 2

The chest gets plenty of work from push-ups, chest presses, and shoulder work, but the upper back tends to be passive unless actively trained. In fact, many of the strength athletes I have worked with have all improved their performance by strengthening their upper backs. Rowing and pulling motions are key for strengthening the upper back, and there are plenty of varieties to try that target different areas. Of course, just practicing good posture with your shoulders back and head up will go a long way as well.

WHAT ARE THE BASICS OF "GOOD FORM?"

The human body is fluid and dynamic and able to move in an infinite number of ways. Dancers and gymnasts are particularly good at showcasing this ability. However, when building strength to reinforce good posture, we want to mimic those postural positions as much as possible in the exercises we do.

The exception to this rule is when strengthening the muscles of the core; we do want to allow for some flexion, extension, and rotation of the spine to specifically strengthen these muscles and their ability to move three dimensions. Otherwise, the alignment of each section of your body should remain relatively constant when performing the majority of any standing exercises such as squats, deadlifts, presses, rows, etc.

With these movements, you must be just as aware of the parts of your body that are providing stability as you are of the parts that are driving the movement. I'm going to give you a few things to think about while performing exercises that will help you make the adjustments you need.

FEET

When you are standing up straight with good posture, you should feel pressure in your feet mostly in your heel to midfoot. That pressure is a cue that indicates whether your center of gravity is correct or not. As I stated above, as soon as you pick up a heavy object, it is going to change the center of gravity of your body. If you start to feel that pressure shift to the front of your foot, that is a cue to adjust your body until that pressure shifts back to the correct position. For example, on an overhead press you may need to lift your chest up whereas on a squat you may need to shift your hips back.

SPINE

The next thing we want to think about is our spine, the area between our hips and our shoulders. Unless we are performing a movement that requires flexion and extension (bending and straightening) of the spine, we want our back to be relatively flat from the top of our shoulders all the way down to our tailbone.

Our upper back is an incredibly important indicator of postural strength. We want to feel that our shoulders are back, and our chest is open and up. This not only engages our back muscles, but it also allows us to breathe more easily. I've noticed that when I instruct new trainees to roll their shoulders back and lift their chests, they often feel a little self-conscious. The truth is, however, they are standing taller with nice upper body carriage and instead of looking floppy and passive, they look strong and capable.

As a whole, we want to see a relatively rigid line from hips to neck whether we are bending our legs or standing straight up. In figure 5.11, Patrick is in the starting position for a deadlift. His back is nice and flat without any excessive rounding of the upper back or inward curvature of the lower back. His head is tilted up, which flexes his neck; this position is fine as it is not affecting his spinal posture. However, some individuals (myself included) have to maintain a neutral neck (so that the spine is straight from head to hips) to prevent inappropriate curvature of the spine.

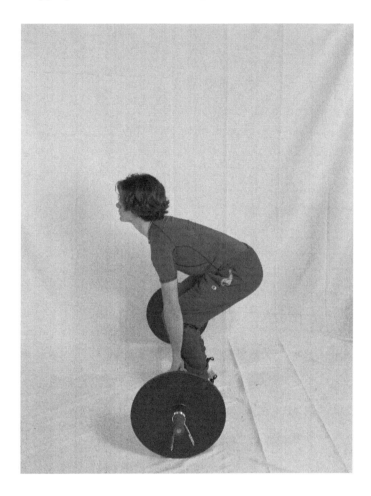

Figure 11: Correct Back Posture

EYES

What are you looking at? Your gaze plays an important role in your ability to execute a movement. In the figure above, Patrick is looking up with both his eyes and his head as he begins his deadlift.

Where you are looking can have a big impact on how you maintain your center of gravity and balance. For example, if trying to balance on one leg, looking straight ahead rather than down greatly increases that ability. Our balance relies on our sight, sensory input from the feet (pressure points from contacting the floor), and neck (which way the head is turned), and the gravity and movement sensors of the inner ear.[114]

As I stated above, some of us can tilt our heads up and down as we move, while others do better if we keep our necks relatively neutral. When teaching the squat to beginners, I encounter a common problem. When the individual tries to keep their gaze forward or up by keeping their chin up (and consequently flexing their neck), it causes excessive curvature of the lower back, as in lordosis. To correct this alignment, I ask them to imagine they are holding a grapefruit or a softball under their chin for the duration of the lift to keep their neck neutral. They can still look up with their eyes without lifting their chins. This technique prevents the lower spine from curving as they bend their hips and legs. In figure 5.12, Shani is looking up with her eyes while keeping her neck neutral on this kettlebell deadlift.

---

114 "The Human Balance System," *Vestibular Disorders Association* (blog), 2016.

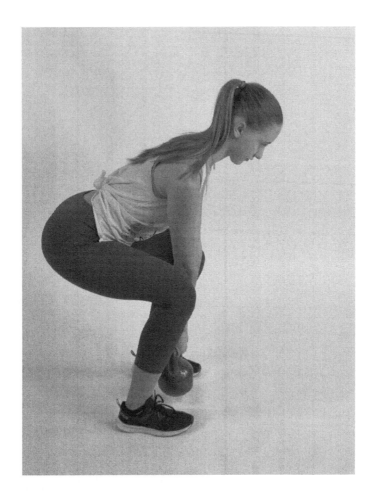

Figure 5.12: Neutral Neck, Looking Up with Eyes

A straight ahead or even upward gaze, regardless of head position, is going to help us keep our balance and maintain our center of gravity when performing standing exercises. Be aware of how your head position may affect your back posture as you move. If flexing or extending your neck negatively affects your back posture, adjust your gaze with eyes only, not your head.

On the other hand, when jumping or doing agility work, it's important that you look where you are stepping or jumping. Especially if you are stepping or jumping on or into an object such as a box or an agility ladder. I have witnessed a number of accidents that could have been easily prevented by simply looking before you leap.

HOW GOOD IS GOOD ENOUGH?

The most important thing to remember is that form is subjective to the individual performing the exercise. An individual's ideal form will be dependent on their abilities and limitations and how much experience they have with the exercise. Expecting a beginner to have perfect form 100 percent of the time is not only unrealistic, but it can also be demoralizing. The goal is to constantly work toward becoming better.

Keep in mind that old injuries, limb length discrepancies, and other deficiencies may not be correctable. In these cases, you will have to determine if you can work around it or if you need a substitute exercise.

THE TOOLS

We can't talk about strength training without talking about our tools for creating resistance. You don't need a fully stocked gym to get strong and fit. However, a few exercises will be more effective if you can add some external resistance such as dumbbells, kettlebells, bars, and/or elastic bands.

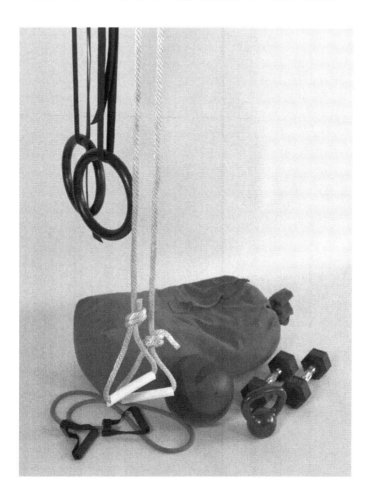

Figure 5.13: Equipment

You can strength train in a number of ways with objects you have around your house or can easily make with a trip to the hardware store. Before we get to the next chapter, think about what sort of equipment you have access to, what you might want to purchase or borrow, or what you can make at home. Here are some things to consider:

RESISTANCE BANDS

Resistance bands encompass a broad range of implements including open-ended surgical tubing and rubber bands with or without handles as well as closed-end bands that can be placed around the feet, knees, or arms. Unlike weighted implements that provide resistance to gravity, resistance bands can provide resistance in multiple directions, mainly depending on where the band is anchored.

Resistance bands can be used with a partner or independently. If you are working in an outdoor space and do not have a place to anchor the bands, having a partner hold the band or lace multiple ones together to provide an anchor allows for a variety of exercises that include rowing, standing presses, and standing pulls. To utilize the bands for upward movements such as squats, deadlifts, and overhead presses, the bands can be anchored by standing on them.

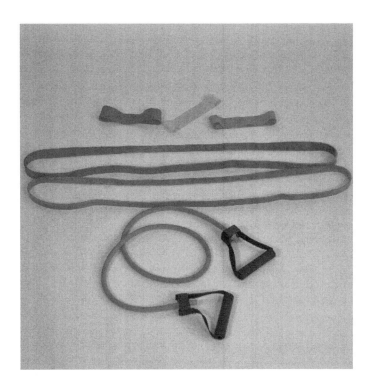

Figure 5.14: Resistance Bands

DUMBBELLS AND KETTLEBELLS

Dumbbells and kettlebells are very versatile and can be used for strength training, muscular endurance training, power training, and general conditioning. Dumbbells and kettlebells come in a broad range of styles. Some are molded or bolted together to remain at a fixed weight, while others are adjustable.

For most beginners, just a few weights are plenty. I usually recommend that you have a set of very light weights, three to five pounds, for rehab exercises (we all need a little rehab) and then two to three heavier weights for your main exercise. These weights can be anywhere from ten to fifty pounds, with the heavier weights being used for heavier loaded exercises such as the deadlift. I will discuss weights more in depth when we talk about specific exercises in the next chapter.

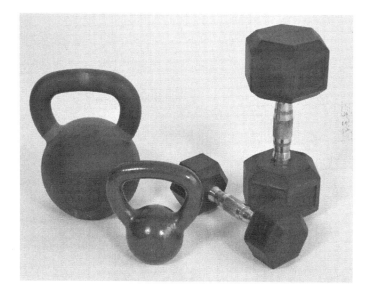

Figure 5.15: Dumbbells and Kettlebells

BARS

Bars and barbells are great tools for building strength. They also have some limitations. For example, if you have shoulder mobility issues, using a bar for squats and presses may restrict movement, so dumbbells or kettlebells may be a better choice.

I love using barbells for deadlifts because this exercise is one lift that we can load relatively heavily, and a bar makes them more ergonomic. I also love using them for barbell complexes, a kind of circuit training where you complete a series of lifts for a prescribed number of repetitions. Once you reach a level of strength and conditioning where you want to include barbell training, I would recommend you reach out to a local strength coach for one-on-one instruction.

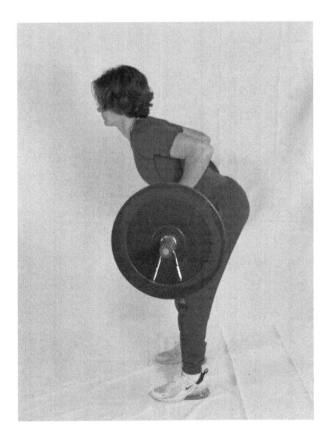

Figure 5.16: Barbell Row

MEDICINE BALLS AND SLAM BALLS

I love medicine balls. These balls typically weigh anywhere from two to twenty pounds, are easy to handle, and usable for pretty much all your exercises. As an implement, medicine balls are extremely versatile and make training with a partner a little more fun. You can use them as resistance for squatting, pressing, or doing sit-ups and rotational movements. You can throw them at a wall, bounce them off the ground, or throw them back and forth with a partner. Between four and eight pounds is typically all most people need to get an effective workout with a medicine ball.

Slam balls are a different kind of medicine ball that are typically filled with sand. These balls are made in much heavier increments than traditional medicine balls. They don't bounce, which means you can throw them, and they won't roll away from you, especially when you are outside. Another DIY solution for a slam ball is to fill an old basketball with sand and then wrap it in duct tape.

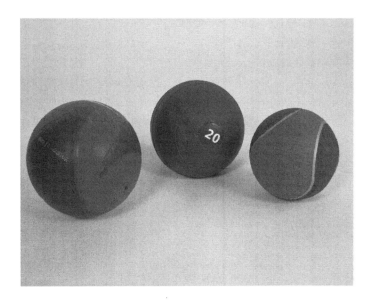

Figure 5.17: Medicine and Slam Balls

ODD OBJECTS FOR STRONGMAN STYLE TRAINING

You don't have to be a strongman to train like one. Strong-man competitions involve lifting, dragging, pulling, and carrying various odd objects such as axles, stones, sandbags, tires, and pretty much anything that might be too heavy or awkward for the average person. However, strongman-style training, scaled to the average person's abilities, is quite beneficial in improving the performance of daily activities. Picking up and carrying heavy and awkward things, bags of mulch, furniture, groceries, children, or dogs is a part of our everyday life whether we like it or not, so we might as well train for it. Proper form and technique are still a priority as these movements require more balance, stability, and core strength than typical gym exercises. Because they are more challenging, lighter weights provide a lot more stimulation to the nervous system.

My favorite strongman tool is a sandbag. Sandbags are extremely versatile and can easily and cheaply be made using army duffle bags and a filler such as wood pellets, rubber mulch, and/or sand. Personally, I would not recommend filling your sandbag with sand unless it is very small. A thirty-five-to-fifty-pound bag is heavy enough for most people, although for smaller adults and children, a twenty-to-thirty-pound bag would be sufficient.

Sandbags can be carried for a distance, used for squats or deadlifts, cleaned and shouldered, and used as a jump platform or obstacle.

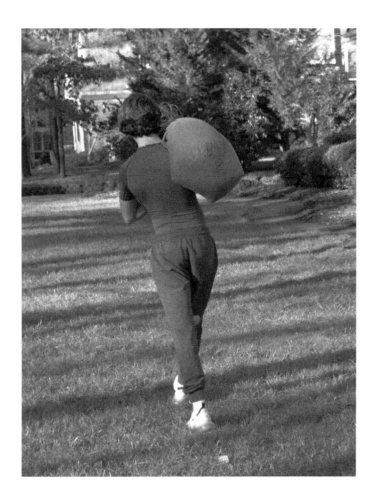

Figure 5.18: Sandbag Carry

PULL-UP BARS AND GYMNASTIC RINGS

Pull-ups and body rows are very effective compound upper body movements that do not require any additional weight. You can also use rings to assist lower body movements such as squats and lunges. Therefore, a pull-up bar and/or some gymnastic rings can be a valuable addition to your home gym. There are many doorway and wall mounted pull-up bars you can purchase. Gymnastic rings can be secured to a wall or door mount or can be hung from your pull-up bar. In figure 5.19, Elizabeth is performing ring rows on rings secured to a ceiling-mounted pull-up bar.

You can easily make a homemade set of gymnastic rings with some polyester rope and some six-inch lengths of one-inch PVC pipe for handles. Just be sure that the method you use to hang or mount them will support your weight. In figure 5.13, a set of homemade rings made from white nylon rope and PVC pipe handles is hanging next to black gymnastic rings.

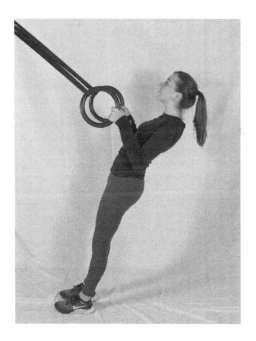

Figure 5.19: Ring Rows

STABILITY BALL

These are those large inflatable balls in multiple colors and sizes that seem to be ubiquitous in every gym. They are a great tool for core exercises like crunches and back extensions and can even be used for hamstring curls. They are also quite comfortable to sit on, and using one as a chair when you are sitting at a desk or table is a great way to train your core and balance while doing other tasks.

BENCH, AEROBIC STEP, OR PLYO BOXES

Many exercises can be modified by raising the height at which you perform it, so having a bench or an aerobic step can be a great addition to your home gym. You can do elevated push-ups, dips, and of course, chest presses from your bench or step. It's also a great tool for bent over rows and core exercises. Plyometric boxes (wooden boxes of varying heights) are a great tool to have as well. You can use these or an aerobic step to perform step ups or even box jumps. Twelve inches is plenty of height for both stepping and jumping.

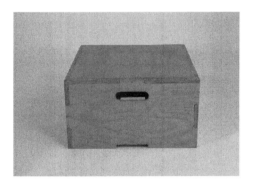

Figure 5.20: Box

PRACTICE MAKES PERFECT

Strength training is important for balanced full-body function, but I want to make one more very important point:

*If you practice your strength training techniques **in your every-day activities**, you will get stronger and more functional every day **by simply living**—no need to spend hours in the gym.*

This means that once you learn to squat properly using your hips, core, and legs, you will use those muscles to get in and out of a sitting position instead of passively dropping or using the momentum or your arms to get up. It means that when you pick up and carry heavy objects, you will be maintaining good posture with your back as you use your legs to lift, and you will stabilize your core. When you walk your dog, your kids, or just yourself, you will be holding your shoulders back, chest up, and abdomen tight, swinging your arms and legs with ease. This change may seem difficult at first, but you will be amazed at how much easier all movement gets in a relatively short amount of time.

It is by committing to using what you learn in the gym in your everyday life that you can spend less time "exercising" and more time actually living.

CHAPTER 6

STRENGTH TRAINING: THE FIRST MOVEMENTS

———

Practicing movement is how we develop strength. Practicing movement against resistance is how we get stronger. In this chapter, you are going to learn how to perform six fundamental movements. You are going to figure out if and how you need to modify each exercise based on your abilities and what equipment you have available. These exercises are the essential movements for those new to training and should be a part of most people's training programs regardless of fitness level. These exercises alone can provide a good strength foundation, and they will also teach you a lot about how the different parts of your body interact with each other to create movement.

HOW TO USE THIS CHAPTER

This chapter is meant to be hands-on, so I want you to approach it a little differently.

1. Read this chapter through once to familiarize yourself with the exercises and what kind of equipment you may want to use.

2. Set aside some time, about forty-five minutes to an hour would be good, to go through this chapter again with the goal of trying out all the exercises and performing the circuits at the end.

3. Be sure to wear loose fitting clothing that doesn't restrict movement.

4. As you try out each exercise, figure out what modifications and additional equipment you need going forward.

5. Record any modifications in your training log.

Remember, this is a learning process, so it's better to start easy and reinforce good movement patterns before moving on to more challenging exercises. I can't tell you how many trainees I've watched completely derail their progress by either refusing to be patient and learn or just not engaging mentally in our training sessions. Instead of "getting it over with," I want you think more about how you are going to win the workout.

"WINNING THE WORKOUT"

I first picked up a copy of Vern Gambetta's book, *Athletic Development*, in February of 2011 at the recommendation of a fellow coach. I had started training my kids and some of their friends, and I was looking for ideas for designing workouts that would be both fun and have some carry-over to whatever sports they were participating in. The book contains practical training advice on everything from what exercises to choose to how to condition different athletes for the demands of their sport. The practical advice was great and helped put a lot of training practices into context; however, a very important aspect of the book was the psychological importance of approaching training with the correct mindset.

One of the core concepts described in this book was the idea of "winning the workout." This surprisingly simple trick is one I still use while training to this day. Gambetta initially heard this concept from swim coach Wayne Goldsmith and describes it in his own words as follows: "Winning the workout consists of high-quality work done with intent and purpose. Remember that quality is a measure of perfect. The goal is always high-quality work coupled with perfect effort looking toward preparation for competition. We always aim to own the finish."[115]

The idea behind this is simple. When we are prescribed a workout, there are several different ways we can go about executing it.

- We can just go through the motions—floppy, apathetic, disinterested in the outcome.
- We can go in with the throttle wide open regardless of the purpose with pain and fatigue as the ultimate goal.

OR

- We can focus on *accumulating a higher volume of good quality work* that will lead to our long-term improvement.

If you recall from Chapter Two, that last bit was the crux of Stephen Seiler's research into polarized training. It is

---

115 Vern Gambetta, "Win the Workout," *HMMR Media* (blog), June 1, 2020.

the high-quality, higher-volume, lower-intensity work that brings the greatest changes. If you want to do it right, think about the purpose of the workout and how you can get the most out of it while doing the least damage. As a trainer and coach, I know that this approach is the most ideal, but is often the most difficult when it comes to getting clients and athletes to follow suit.

WARMING UP

Before you begin, it's always a good idea to warm up to get your blood flowing and your muscles more pliable. You can do this any number of ways: go for a walk, jog in place, do some calisthenics such as jumping jacks, toe touches, etc. I usually have my trainees warm up by moving all the joints in the body in multiple directions starting with the spine.

This is a good warm-up routine that addresses pretty much everything and only takes about five minutes to complete. Complete each exercise ten times:

	Body Part	Instructions
Toe Touches	Spine	With knees slightly bent, slowly bend down, one vertebrate at a time, until your fingers can touch your feet (or somewhere below the knee), and then slowly rise back up. Try to increase range of motion with each repetition.
Shoulder Rotation	Spine	Raise up your arms and put your elbows out to the side. With slightly bent knees, rotate your shoulders perpendicular to your hips back and forth to both sides. Do this relatively swiftly and try to get as much range of motion as possible. Placing a broomstick or length of PVC pipe behind your back will help open your chest and maintain your posture.
Side Bends	Spine	Standing straight up, bend to your left and then reverse and bend to your right. Again, using a broomstick or length of PVC pipe to lock your arms overhead will help maintain your posture.
Knee Hugs	Hips and Hamstrings	You can do these exercises while standing, sitting, or lying on your back, but standing will require some balance. Lift one knee and quickly hug it as close to your chest as possible with your arms. Switch legs and do the same with the other. Do these relatively quickly as though marching in place.
Quad Stretches	Quads	These stretches are easier if you can hold onto a wall or stabilize yourself with a broomstick. Keeping your thigh straight down, you want to bend your knee and lift your ankle and grab it with your hand and stretch. If you can't quite reach, use a strap to pull your foot up toward your back.
Shoulder Circles	Shoulders	I find these exercises get more range of motion when you do one arm at a time. Stretch your arm out and rotate it around your shoulder joint in as big a circle as you can. Do ten rotations in each direction and then switch arms.
Ankle Stretch: Heel/Toe Walk	Calves/Shins	Stabilize yourself by holding onto a wall or broomstick. In a marching-in-place fashion, alternate stepping up onto your toes and then down onto your heels while pointing your toes up. Alternatively, you can alternate stepping on your heels and toes as you walk back and forth for ten steps each direction.

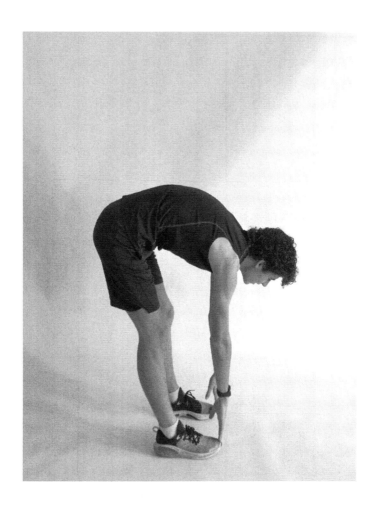

Figure 6.1: Toe Touches

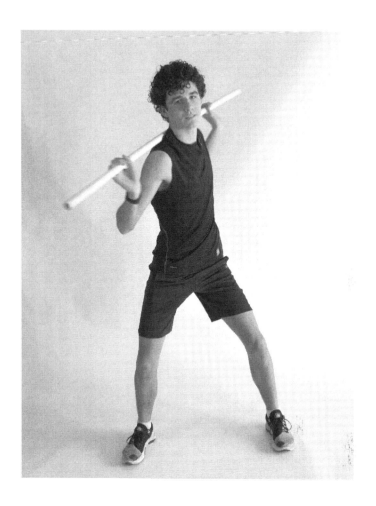

Figure 6.2: Shoulder Rotation

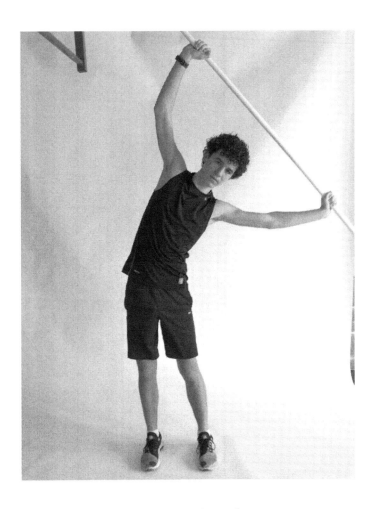

Figure 6.3: Side Bends

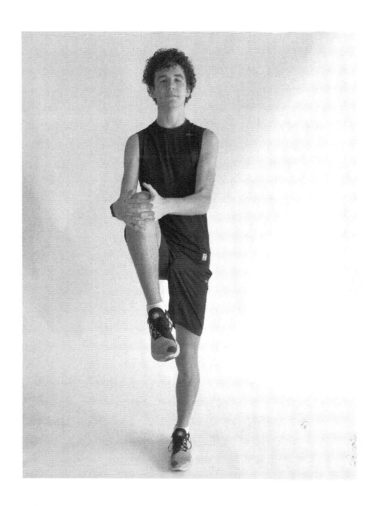

Figure 6.4: Knee Hugs

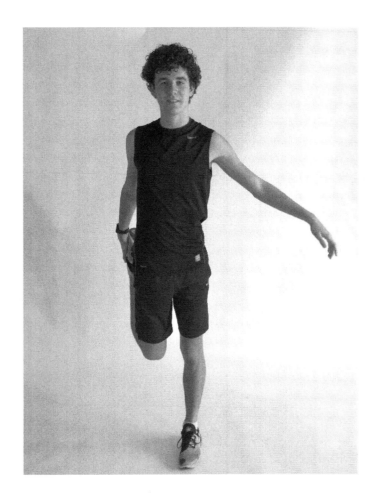

Figure 6.5: Quad Stretches

HOW TO CHECK YOUR FORM

To perform strength exercises correctly, observation is key. For this reason, I highly recommend using a mirror or even taking video of your movements to make sure your form is correct. I use video or someone else's eyes semi-regularly to keep me on track when it comes to my form and technique. There is always room for improvement.

Here is a short summary of the form guidelines given in Chapter Five, which you can refer to when checking your form on the exercises that follow. Start with the simplest form of the exercise that you think you can perform well and go from there.

Form Checklist:

- Where are your feet positioned?
- How is your posture?
- Where are you looking?
- What is the primary goal of the movement?
- What parts of your body are moving?
- What parts of your body are stable?

Possible Issues:

- Does the starting position or movement cause you any pain?
- Do you have any issues maintaining your balance?
- Are there any limitations to your range of motion?
- What parts of your form break down as you fatigue?

Solutions:

- What adjustments can you make to mitigate pain or discomfort?
- What is your current comfortable range of motion?

- What cues can you use to remind yourself about form breakdown during a movement?

THE FIRST MOVEMENTS

I use six basic exercises to both evaluate my clients and start building their strength. As I am teaching them, I am personalizing and modifying each exercise for their individual starting point. These modified versions become the foundational movements of their initial training program.

I use these exercises because together, they address the major muscle groups and movement patterns of the body. They are highly effective at building strength and improving function. As my clients improve, I make the exercises more challenging by increasing range of motion, adding resistance, using different tools, and/or adding more variety to their workouts. However, this is the starting point for everyone: **squat, push-up, row, deadlift, press, rotation**.

THE SQUAT

The squat is probably the most important strength-building exercise we can do for several reasons.

- Squats strengthen most of the major muscles of the lower body and core.
- Squatting enables us to practice that important skill of getting up from a sitting position, something that quite a few people lose with age.
- Squats involve bending the knees and hips while externally rotating the knee, an important movement for

strengthening the gluteus medius, the muscle that stabilizes our knee when walking or running.

Personally, as I've gotten older and knee pain has begun to creep into my life, squatting regularly helps keep it at bay.

How to Squat

The squat is a complex movement that is easily learned if you keep a few basic concepts in mind. We want to begin by getting our feet in the right position. Feet should be somewhere between hip and shoulder width apart with the toes turned slightly out. In figure 6.6 you can see the foot position as Elizabeth initiates her squat. Her knees track out in line with her toes as she squats, and her thighs are parallel with her feet. Elizabeth's squat stance is relatively wide because she has long legs relative to her torso. Due to differences in the structures of our hip bones and pelvis, individuals require different stance widths and toe positions to squat comfortably. These stances may change as they get stronger and more flexible.

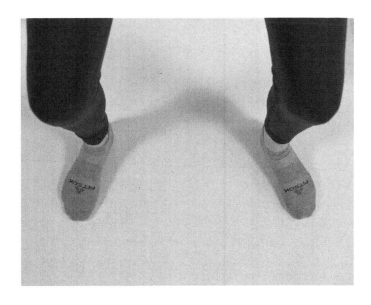

Figure 6.6: Squat Knee and Toe Position

The next thing to be aware of is where your center of gravity is. As we discussed in Chapter Five, an easy clue is where you feel pressure in your feet as you squat. Ideally, you should feel pressure somewhere between your midfoot and heel. If you feel pressure in the ball of your foot or toes, your center of gravity is too far forward.

The reason I bring this topic up is that in new squatters, the most common fault is to begin the squat by bending the knees forward. This action may not bother some people, but it puts some unideal pressure on the knee joint and causes pain and injury over time. In general, the knees should not go any further forward than the toes. To initiate the squat correctly, you want to first get your feet into the correct position and begin by pushing your hips back behind you. In figure

6.7, Shani has initiated this first squat by bending her knees forward. As you can see, squatting this way results in her barely reaching the front of the chair behind her. In figure 6.8, she is initiating her squat by pushing her hips back first, and in figure 6.9 you can see that this movement results in a squat that allows her to sit farther back on the chair.

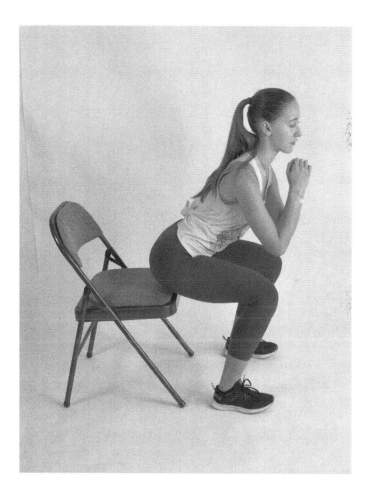

Figure 6.7: Forward Squat

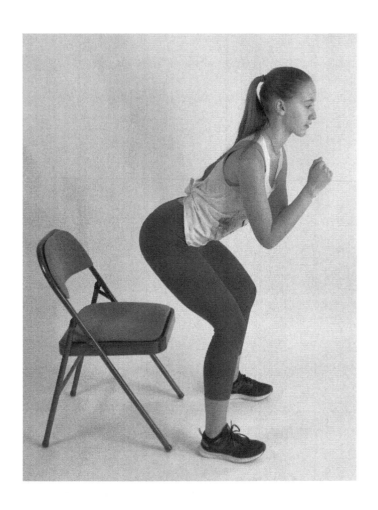

Figure 6.8: Hips Back

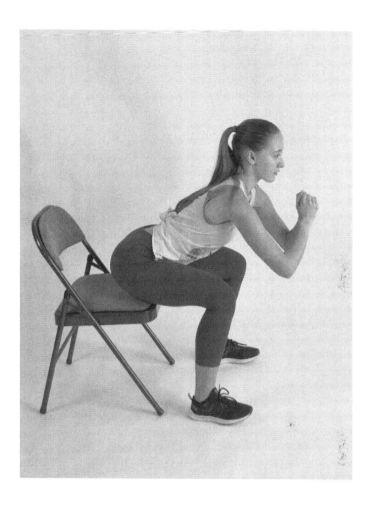

Figure 6.9: More Perfect Squat

It is perfectly okay to lean forward to balance yourself as you squat. In fact, this is a tactic you can use to get up from a chair without rocking or pushing yourself up with your arms. Leaning forward helps to balance your center of gravity while pushing your hips behind you. Individuals with long legs often have a more forward leaning squat than individuals with short legs. As long as you maintain your straight back posture, there can be lot of variability in the angle of your back relative to the floor (more forward or more upright).

Pushing your hips farther behind you as you squat can make some people feel as though they are going to lose their balance and fall back, so I always have my beginners squat to a chair or a box. If you find you are still uneasy with your balance, hold a light weight out in front of you as you squat. Again, this will help shift your center of gravity forward so you can push your hips back further. In figure 6.10, Shani is holding a medicine ball to help her balance while pushing her hips behind her. This kind of squat is known as a goblet squat, as if you were holding a goblet out in front of you with both hands.

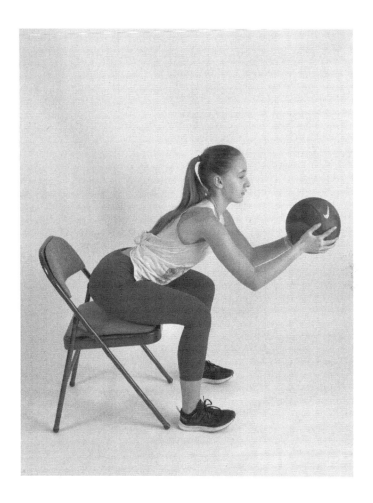

Figure 6.10: Medicine Ball Squat

Set-up

1. Place a chair or a box behind you at a height you feel comfortable with.
2. Stand directly in front of the chair, about six inches away from the seat.

3. Stand with your feet about shoulder-distance apart. (Standing in front of a mirror will help you judge your stance width more accurately.)
4. Turn your toes slightly out, maybe twenty to thirty degrees, as shown in figure 6.6.

Execution

1. To begin the squat, push your hips back and reach for the back of the chair with your rear.
2. As you descend, be conscious of pushing your knees out to stay in line with your toes. You may need to lean forward and/or reach forward with your arms to keep your balance.
3. As soon as your bottom touches the chair, keep your muscles engaged and try to reverse the movement by driving up with your hips and legs.*

If you get to the chair and find you can't reverse the movement, place a thick book or even a cushion on the chair to give you a higher target. The goal of having the chair behind you is not to sit down, it is to simply give you a stopping place for depth and also catch you if you lose your balance. This height can gradually be lowered or removed altogether as you become stronger.

The important thing to remember here is that we are trying to activate the muscles of the hips. Try to refrain from doing things like rocking up out of the chair or swinging your arms in order to get back up. If that is something you feel you have to do, then I would prefer that you actually lean forward or pick up a weight and hold it in front of you. This will shift your center of gravity forward and that's going to help you get up out of that chair without having to use any excess momentum.

Proper squatting form is heavily debated, and one of the most argued-about points is how deep to squat. Some people believe a deep squat is important, and in certain ways they are correct in that it is difficult to avoid using your hips when squatting with your hips below your knees. However, deeper squats can disproportionately increase stress on the knees, so we need to be careful about adding resistance while increasing range of motion.[116]

For most healthy people, squatting with your hips back until the top of your thighs are parallel to the floor is plenty of depth. If you have trouble getting that low, no worries, as long as you are reaching back with your hips, you will eventually get there with practice. Adjusting the width of your stance or pointing your toes and knees out more may help as well. The structure of your pelvis will dictate your ideal squat form so try a few different stance widths and toe angles if you are having trouble getting your hips back and down.

Once you can squat easily to a chair and get back up, try it without the chair and see if you can squat freely without going forward into your knees. Some people will always want to squat to a chair or a box and that's fine. In fact, many of my strength athletes routinely squat to a box to help with

---

116 Joshua A. Cotter et al., "Knee Joint Kinetics in Relation to Commonly Prescribed Squat Loads and Depths," *Journal of Strength and Conditioning Research / National Strength & Conditioning Association* 27, no. 7 (July 2013): 1769–7.

consistency of depth, especially when our training sessions have a lot of repetitions.

There are many ways we can add resistance to a squat. In figure 6.11, Shani is squatting with a light bar on her back. This version of the squat requires flexible shoulders and an open chest, and it is particularly helpful for enhancing upper back strength in addition to leg, hip, and core strength.

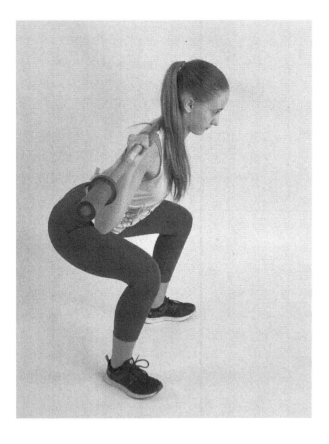

Figure 6.11: Squat with Bar

In figure 6.12, Francis is performing a goblet squat with a kettlebell. This squat is particularly helpful if you have trouble getting your hips back without a chair or box behind you. You can perform this with virtually any implement you can hold in front of you.

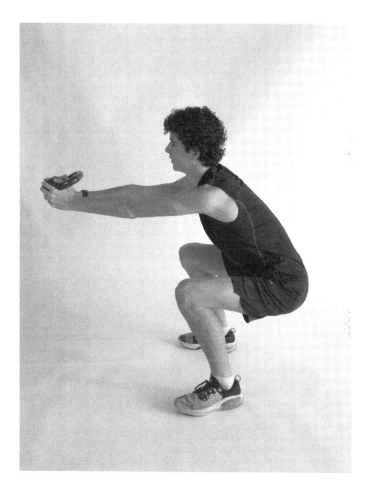

Figure 6.12: Goblet Squat

In figure 6.13, Francis is performing a back squat with a barbell. The barbell back squat is a version of the squat that can be loaded with a great deal of weight. The bar is placed on your upper back, just above the shoulder blades, so this version of the lift requires shoulder flexibility and a strong back and core. Typically, this is performed with a rack to hold the bar between sets. Because the weights are significantly heavier than what you can lift off the floor and place on your back, these can easily compromise your form and posture. If you reach the point where you want to add more weight to your squat, I highly recommend finding a local coach who can safely instruct you in person until you can perform this lift consistently and with good form.

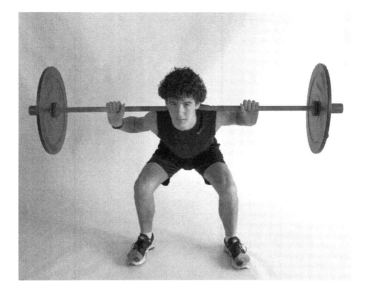

Figure 6.13 Barbell Back Squat

To get started with squatting, you want to find a version of which you can perform ten to fifteen repetitions easily, with good form, and without any pain in your knees or hips. Use a mirror or video camera to check your stance and your posture. Figure out what tools (chair, dumbbell, etc.) you need to perform your squat correctly and consistently and make a note in your training log. As you get better at squatting, you can adjust your depth, your resistance, and the number of sets and reps you can do.

THE PUSH-UP

Push-ups may seem like an exercise that only fitness buffs and military types do, but this versatile exercise is easily modifiable, meaning that people of any level can do them. The push-up is a great exercise for the upper body as well as the core. It requires that you stabilize the muscles of your abdomen and lower back (your core muscles) while using your shoulders, arms, and chest to raise and lower your body. Push-ups can be done virtually anywhere and don't require any equipment.

How to do a Push-up

The set-up for a push-up is to get into a plank position with your hands on the floor (or a raised surface) under your shoulders. If you are doing push-ups off a raised surface such as a bench or a countertop, your hands may be further down your chest when you are in the bottom position. The width of your hands can be adjusted for comfort. Your legs can be supported by either your knees or your toes.

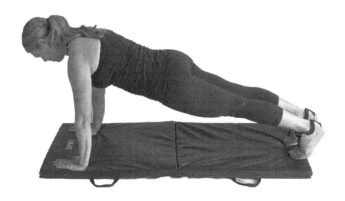

Figure 6.14: Push-up Set-up

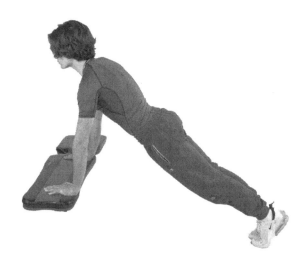

Figure 6.15: Push-up from Bench

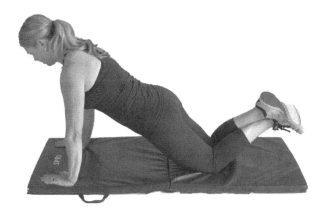

Figure 6.16: Push-up from Knees

The most important part of the push-up is the stability of your trunk. Your back should not sink down as in figure 6.17 or arch up as in figure 6.18. Instead, we should see a nice straight line from your head to your hips.

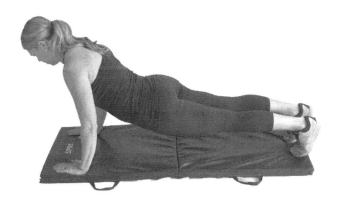

Figure 6.17: Back Sunk

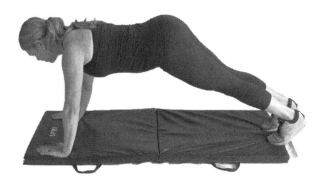

Figure 6.18: Back Arched

The first modification I make for individuals who either can't keep their core stable or simply can't push themselves up off the floor is to either raise the surface on which they place their hands (you can use a bench or countertop), or have the individual perform the push-up from their knees. Some coaches and trainers object to knee push-ups. I think there is absolutely nothing wrong with them as long as the individual keeps their body in a straight line from knees to neck as in figure 6.16. This is an easy way for them to build core and upper body strength until we can increase the resistance by having them go to their toes or lowering the surface they are pushing up from.

Set-up and Execution

* Obviously, if you aren't sure whether or not you can do a push-up off the floor, there is no harm in trying. You might surprise yourself.

1. Get into a plank position as shown in figure 6.14 with your hands under your shoulders. Some people prefer a wider or narrower grip; it's up to your individual comfort.
2. Make sure your low back is not sagging, as in figure 6.17, by pulling your belly button in toward your spine.
3. Ensure your butt is not sticking up as in figure 6.18. This prevents you from engaging your core muscles properly.
4. Lower yourself down until your chest is just above the floor (or raised surface) and then, keeping your core tight, push yourself back up.

If you can't do a full push-up, or can only do a few, no worries—practice makes perfect. If completing ten repetitions is difficult, try doing more sets of smaller numbers of reps. For example, eight sets of three to five reps. The outcome will still be the same number of recommended total reps, but it's just broken into smaller sets. If you can do a small number of full push-ups, start with those, then complete your set of ten with whatever modification you prefer. Going to your knees is the easiest in my opinion as you don't have to move mid-set. With practice, you will be able to increase your numbers over time. Record what modifications you used in your training log.

THE ROW

Rowing movements are extremely important for upper back strength. A lack of upper back strength can result in rounded posture, especially in desk workers, and eventual remodeling of the spine. Rowing is simply the act of pulling something toward you and includes all kinds of movements such as the barbell row shown in figure 6.19, bench row as shown in figure 6.21, pull-ups, and ring rows as shown in figure 6.23. Even working out on a rowing machine can help build upper back strength.

Rowing can be done with any kind of exercise equipment, resistance bands, or even your own bodyweight. Rowing activates most of the large muscle groups of the upper back as well as the arms. As we have discussed, upper back weakness is a key contributor to bad posture, so rows should be an essential part of your training program. I am going to give you three different ways to perform this exercise. Choose the one that works best for you.

Set-up and Execution

In figure 6.19, Patrick is demonstrating perfect form for the **standing row**. You can perform this with a bar or with a set of dumbbells or kettlebells.

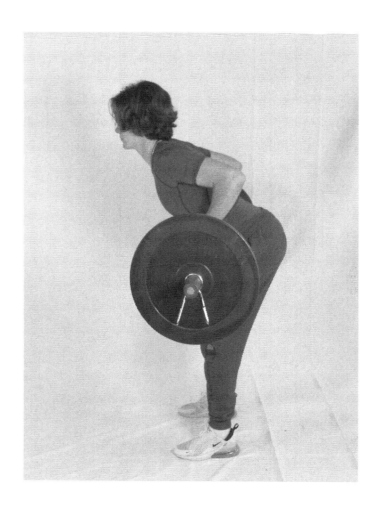

Figure 6.19: Standing Row Top Position

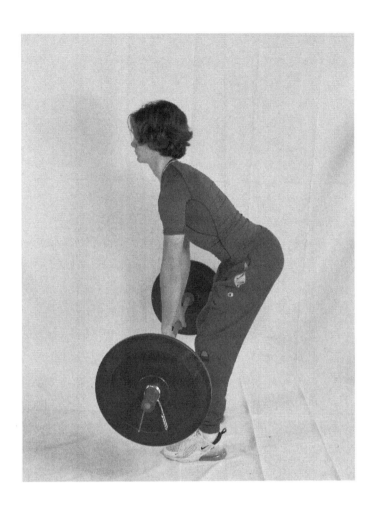

Figure 6.20: Standing Row Bottom Position

1. Begin by holding the weight(s) in both hands with your feet directly below your hips, toes pointed forward.
2. Push your hips back behind you, as in the squat, keeping your weight in your heels and bending your knees slightly until the bar (or other implement) reaches knee height as in figure 6.20.

3. Your back should be straight from hips to neck, and your shoulders should be pulled back with an open chest.
4. Pull your belly button in to your spine to prevent excessive curvature of the low back.
5. To execute the lift, simply pull your elbows straight back, as if you are pulling straight into your belly button.

A **bench row** is a good option for individuals who have a hard time keeping their backs straight when executing this lift. This exercise is typically performed with a dumbbell or kettlebell, and you are only working one side at a time. A bench is ideal for this exercise. Two chairs or stools of the same height can be easily substituted. The idea is to support the hand and knee of the inactive side with the bench, which enables the individual to form a "table" with their back. On the active side, the leg is on the floor and the arm lowers the weight below the height of the bench. Don't let the back become passive and sag down when lowering the weight. Rigid posture is an essential part of this exercise.

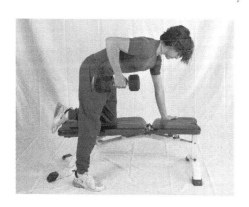

Figure 6.21: Bench Row Top Position

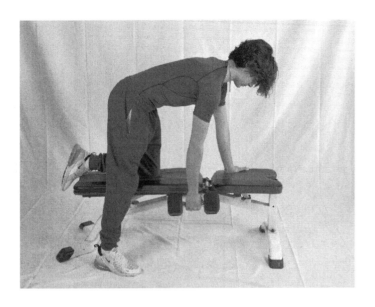

Figure 6.22: Bench Row Bottom Position

The **body or ring row** is like a reverse push-up in that it requires not just arm and upper back engagement, but core stability. If you have something to anchor a set of rings, a suspension apparatus such as a TRX, or even a rope with handles, this row is an easy exercise to incorporate. Adjusting the length of the strap/rope and changing your foot position can make this exercise easier or more difficult. Basically, the further back you can lean, the more force you have to exert to pull yourself up. In figures 6.23 and 6.24, Elizabeth is performing body rows with gymnastic rings attached to a pull-up bar.

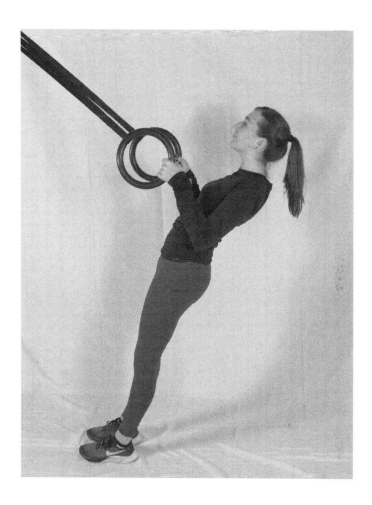

Figure 6.23: Ring Row Top Position

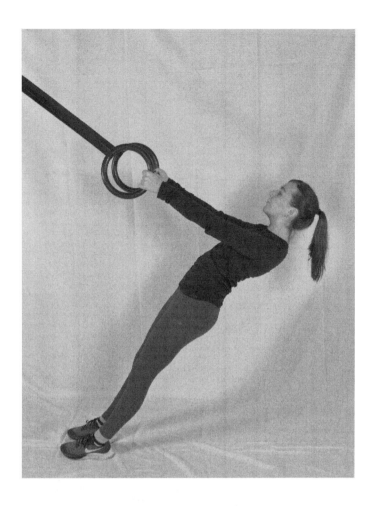

Figure 6.24: Ring Row Bottom Position

THE DEADLIFT

The deadlift is important to pretty much everything in your life. It is what you do any time you pick up something heavy. Deadlifting correctly reduces the amount of force on the spine and distributes it more evenly among the muscles of the legs, core, and hips. We all know someone who threw out their back trying to move heavy furniture or playing with their kids. Sometimes, these injuries are out of our control, but knowing how to deadlift correctly will help prevent most of them.

The deadlift is a different movement from the squat; however, they can look very similar depending on your limb and torso lengths. People with shorter legs—where their femurs and calves are the same length—typically squat and deadlift very similarly whereas people with longer legs tend to bend forward more at the hip when they deadlift.

When picking up everyday objects, most of us are going to squat down and pick up something that is between our feet or slightly in front of us. Therefore, the first way I teach people to deadlift is with a single weight, typically a kettlebell or dumbbell.

Kettlebell or Dumbbell Deadlift

To begin, you will be holding a weight in front of you with both hands. Start with your feet between hip and shoulder width apart with your toes pointed slightly outward.

You will initiate the movement by pushing your hips back behind you and bending your knees as you bend forward and lower the weight down between your feet. You're going to want to keep your back nice and straight from the base of your spine all the way to your neck. How far you lower the weight is up to you, and again, depends on what you can comfortably achieve. Eventually, we would like to see a full range of motion, i.e., touch the object you are holding to the ground.

As you lower the weight, keep it as close to your center as possible. A common fault is to bend your knees forward without pushing the hips back. This will tip you forward and can make your back round. You will counter this tip by continuing to push your hips back as you bend your knees. Keep your shoulders back and your chest open. A little rounding of the upper back is not bad, especially with heavier weights. Rounding of the lower back, however, is very, very bad. We want to avoid that at all costs, as it can do some damage to your lumbar spine.

In figure 6.25, Patrick begins with a kettlebell held in front of his body. As he lowers the kettlebell to the floor, he pushes his hips back such that the kettlebell stays in line vertically with its original position as in figure 6.26. Once his hips are pushed back as far as possible, he begins to bend his knees until the weight is lowered to the floor. As you can see in figure 6.27, the kettlebell is in line with his midfoot and therefore his center of gravity. His back remains straight, his chest is open, and his shoulders are back throughout the whole lift.

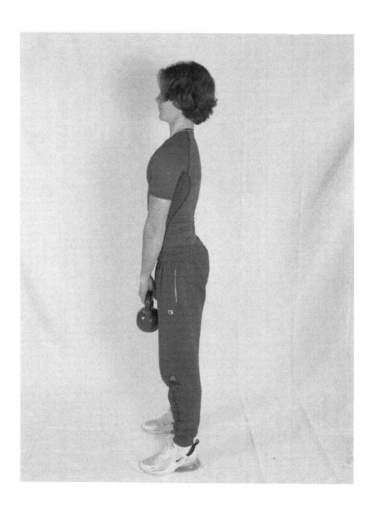

Figure 6.25: Kettlebell Deadlift Top Position

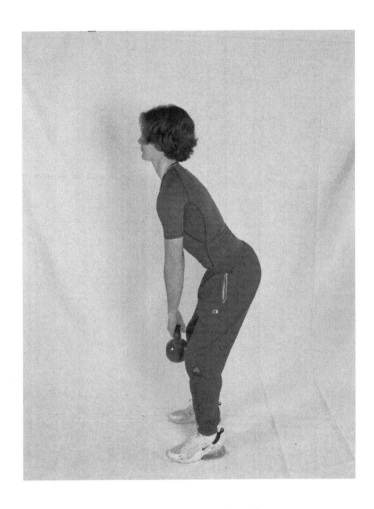

Figure 6.26: Kettlebell Deadlift Mid Position

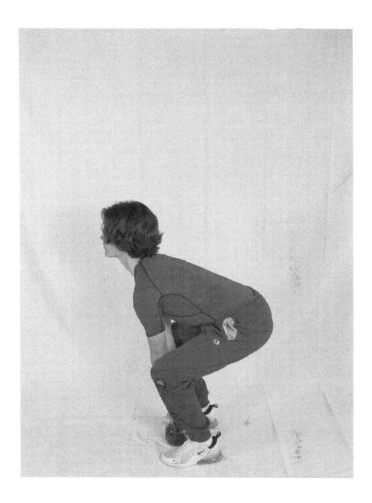

Figure 6.27: Kettlebell Deadlift Bottom Position

When performing this lift, pay attention to the position of
the weight as it approaches the floor. I will often mark an X
between my clients' feet so that they pay attention to where
they are lowering it. Often, as they are focused on different
aspects of the lift, they forget to push their hips back, causing
the weight to drift forward.

Set-up and Execution

1. Begin by holding the weight in both hands with your feet directly below your hips, toes pointed forward.
2. Push your hips back behind you, as in the squat, keeping your weight in your heels and bending your knees slightly until the weight reaches knee height as in figure 6.26.
3. Your back should be straight from hips to neck, and your shoulders should be pulled back with an open chest.
4. Pull your belly button in to your spine to prevent excessive curvature of the low back.
5. Continue to lower the weight by bending your knees until it reaches the floor. If your back starts to curve, you may want to stop at a place higher up, such as where the weight is in line with your mid-shin.
6. Make sure that the weight is not drifting forward as you lower it.
7. Reverse the direction of the lift by first straightening the knees and then pushing the hips forward.

Deadlifting a Bar

The deadlift, like the squat, is another lift that you can load quite a bit when using a bar. If you wish to lift more weight, a barbell is a far more effective tool. Again, I would advise you to work with a coach who can observe and correct your form as you go.

The form principles for a barbell deadlift are very similar to the kettlebell deadlift above. The weight must be as close to your center of gravity as possible (therefore wear knee socks or pants so you don't rub your skin off on the bar.) You must keep your back straight from neck to hips. Your chest should be open, shoulders back, and you want to keep your weight in your heels. Setting up for a barbell deadlift requires that you start at the bottom, so you should feel comfortable getting your hips back behind you in a low position before giving this a try.

Set-up and Execution

1. Step up to the bar such that it is in contact with your shins.
2. Grasp the bar about a thumb's length outside of your legs.
3. Push your hips back and bend your knees until your back is flat and your chest is open as in figure 6.28. Do NOT begin this lift with a rounded back. You should feel tension in your hamstrings.
4. Keeping your upper back tight, pull the bar up your shins by straightening your knees as in figure 6.29.
5. As the bar passes over your kneecap, begin to push your hips forward until you are standing up straight, as in figure 6.30.
6. Reverse the movement to lower the bar back to the floor.

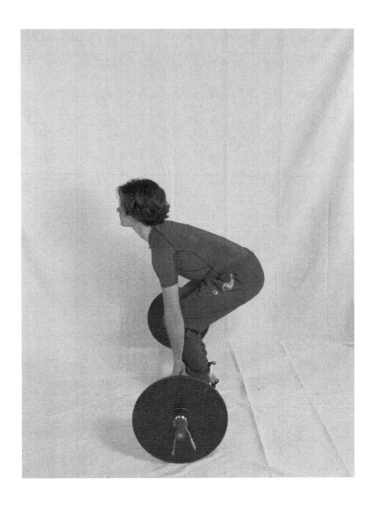

Figure 6.28: Barbell Deadlift Start

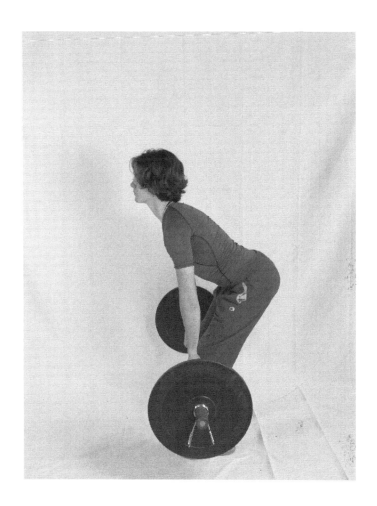

Figure 6.29: Barbell Deadlift Mid-lift

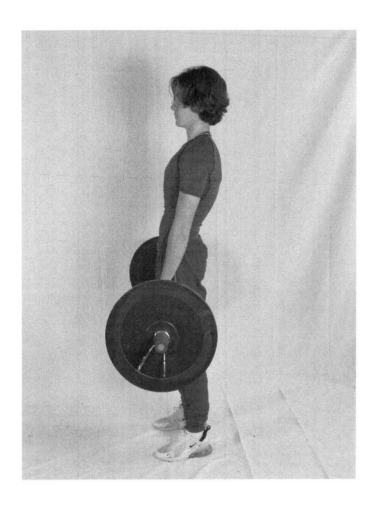

Figure 6.30: Barbell Deadlift Finish

THE PRESS

The overhead press is a movement that I believe is essential for maintaining shoulder function. It is also vital to upper body strength as it targets the shoulders, arms, chest, upper back, and core. Being able to reach overhead and take an object off a high shelf either at home or the store is something we need to be able to do regularly and pressing is a way we can practice this movement with good technique. However, I have had a good number of people who have been told not to press overhead due to arthritis, injury, or pain come to my gym. Sometimes, this advice is given with good reason, especially if the movement causes pain. However, this limitation doesn't mean that the press shouldn't exist in some form or another in your workouts.

To perform the overhead press safely and without pain, there are just a few crucial steps to keep in mind.

The first is simply to keep in mind the principles of good posture: shoulders back, chest open and up, pull your belly button in to your spine, and push your hips forward. Then, simply see if you can raise your arms above your head such that your upper arm is in line with your ear while maintaining that posture. This is a good starting place to evaluate if you have any mobility limitations in performing this movement.

If you have a hard time lifting your arms overhead while standing, it is perfectly acceptable to perform this exercise while seated as well. Some people feel pressure on their lower back when performing overhead movements and sitting can help take that pressure off. You can sit on a bench or even sit in a chair with some back support. If you are seated, don't allow yourself to become passive. Engaged postural muscles are still necessary to fully activate all the upper body muscles involved in this exercise.

The second way to optimize the overhead press is to pay attention to how your wrists are positioned when performing the press. This positioning can make a big difference in how your shoulders feel and how much range of motion you have. You can use a pronated grip, where you have your palms facing away from you, or you can use a neutral grip, where your palms are facing each other. Some people will begin with pronated grip and rotate into a neutral grip as they press and vice versa. This is perfectly fine, do what you find most comfortable for your shoulders.

If you cannot completely extend your arms overhead, that's okay. For some people, it is easier if they only raise one arm at a time. You can modify the angle of the press by leaning into the back of a chair while seated. This version is more of an incline press, which you can eventually work toward getting fully overhead. As long as the weights stay centered over your shoulder, you are fine. Begin with very light weights and work on increasing that range of motion over time. If range of motion or pain continues to be a problem, you may need to seek the advice of a physical therapist.

Set-up and Execution

* *I recommend that everyone begin overhead pressing with dumbbells, kettlebells, or even a set of soup cans or water bottles rather than a bar. A bar doesn't allow for free movement of the shoulder and will lock you into a pronated grip position and a fixed grip width. This position can irritate the shoulder joint over time and cause an overuse injury if not done correctly.*

1. Stand with good posture. Be especially cognizant of your lower back posture. Pull your belly button in toward your spine and push your hips forward. Your feet should be under your hips.
2. Hold your weights up at your shoulders as close to your body as possible and press them overhead ending with your upper arm in line with and next to your ear as in figure 6.31. You can press both at the same time or press them one at a time.
3. Then simply press them overhead with the goal being to get your upper arm in line with your ear. Your weights should be centered over your shoulder joint, not out to the side or out in front. A little bit of deviation is okay, but this exercise is something you can work on improving over time.

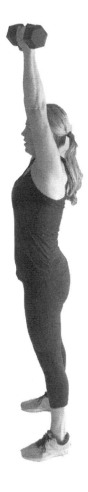

Figure 6.31: Overhead Press Side View

This is a good exercise to perform in front of a mirror as it will require you to keep your eyes forward, enabling you to see the positioning of the weights as well as the relative symmetry of your left and right arm.

ROTATION

Sit-ups and crunches are the most common exercises people think about when training their abdominal muscles. These exercises are actually pretty low down on my list of priorities when it comes to training the core. As you can see, pretty much all the exercises we have gone through so far involve a great deal of core activation for stabilization. Any postural issues you will encounter using those exercises will be primarily the result of weak core muscles.

Controlling the rotation of our hips and shoulders is something we do every day. Rolling over in bed, moving an object from one side to another, and even simply walking all require rotation control. Rotation control has two components: One is actively rotating the shoulders relative to the hips, i.e., twisting your upper body. The other is stabilizing our spine against unintended rotation from poor movement patterns or uneven loads. An example of this misalignment is when you pick up a heavy object with one hand (such as a bucket of water) and your body naturally rotates to maintain your center of gravity. However, it is difficult to walk with a water bucket hanging in front of you so you would engage your core muscles, which prevents that from happening, and keep the water to the side.

Both rotational movements and stability are largely controlled by our obliques, and they also involve our transversus abdominis. The transversus is one of the deep core muscles that Pilates instructors are obsessive about, and for good reason—it's basically the internal corset that protects our lower back and flattens our bellies. The easiest way to start training our core's muscles to control rotation, in my opinion, is standing core work with a medicine ball or some other kind of weight.

Set-up and Execution

*To execute a standing Russian twist, you need a weight of some kind. A ball, a plate, a dumbbell, a kettlebell, or even a brick are all appropriate.

1. Stand with good posture holding your weight in front of you. Your upper arms will be down at your sides and your forearms will be out in front of you at a ninety-degree angle.
2. Soften your knees slightly and keeping your hips facing forward, rotate your upper body to one side as far as you can comfortably go.
3. Immediately reverse the movement all the way to the other side.
4. Be sure to keep your back straight, your hips forward, and your knees soft. Your head should remain in line with your shoulders during the movement as in figure 6.32.

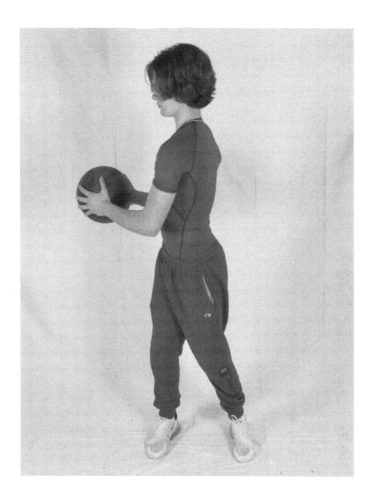

Figure 6.32: Russian Twist with Medicine Ball

YOUR FIRST WORKOUTS

The first couple of times a new client comes to my gym, we stick to these six exercises to find their ideal form, modifications, and resistance. I keep the workouts relatively simple so they don't have to overthink anything, and if they are able to add more sets, reps, or resistance, we do that as we go.

Once you have tried all these exercises out on their own and feel you have a good place to start with each one, I would like you to perform the following two circuits. Ideally, you will do these circuits on different days. If you aren't used to doing these movements, you may be pretty sore no matter how active you usually are. If you aren't sore, that's okay. There's no sense in crippling yourself your first week in. If you complete your circuit and still feel like you can do more, go for a walk.

Circuit 1: Squat, Push-up, Row

Circuit 2: Deadlift, Press, Rotation

To perform these circuits, you are going to set a goal of three to five rounds of ten to fifteen reps per set of exercise. The exception to this rule will be on push-ups and presses, where five to ten repetitions will be the goal if ten to fifteen is out of reach for now.

For the sake of using common terms going forward, let me explain a little more clearly. "Reps" refers to how many repetitions of a single exercise you do at once. If you start squatting and did eight squats before you stopped to rest, that would be eight reps.

If the only exercise you were doing was squats and you rested after a certain number of reps before doing more, all of your groups of repetitions together are referred to as a "set." In single exercise training, you will perform multiple sets of a single exercise.

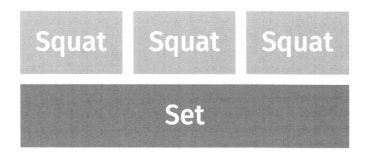

When we are doing more than one exercise at a time, i.e., we are going to do a certain number of squats, then push-ups, then rows before starting over again with squats, the group of repetitions for each complete set of exercises is called a "round." In circuit training, you will perform multiple rounds of each group of exercises.

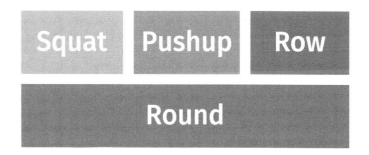

THE IMPORTANCE OF REST PERIODS

Resting between each set or each round is not only good, but I would also encourage you to do so whenever you feel the need. If you try to push through a workout without rest, you will fatigue early and be unable to ***accumulate the volume of good quality work*** that is necessary to improve. (I realize this phrase is getting repetitive, but this is the most important part of training.)

At first, you may rest until you feel ready to begin again. As you become more conditioned, you will want to limit your rest periods to no more than one to two minutes. Eventually you will want to complete all the exercises in a single round before resting. For now, if you need to rest after each exercise, that's fine.

If you find you are needing to rest more often and for longer periods, you need to lessen the intensity or difficulty of the exercise. Decrease weight, reduce range of motion, do whatever you have to do in order to complete your reps without discomfort.

Complete fatigue is the enemy of progress. We want to feel like we worked, but burning and fatigued muscles are not the end game here. Not only do you want to accumulate high-quality volume, but you also want to be able to function for the remainder of your day without needing to take a nap on your desk or be unable to get out of your chair.

WINNING THIS WORKOUT

To win this workout, you are going to focus on four things:

1. Learn how to repeat the movements consistently. You may have to actively think about keeping your core tight on push-ups or pushing your knees out to stay in line with

your feet on squats. Remember these cues and record them in your training log.

2. Figure out how much resistance to use. You may start with no weight and realize the exercise is far too easy. Likewise, you may start with a weight and realize that you are unable to complete the prescribed number of repetitions. At first, it is okay to increase or decrease your resistance from round to round or even mid-set. Once you find your groove, you want to work with small increases over time so you can continue to make progress.

3. Figure out what range of motion is comfortable for you. As you complete more repetitions of an exercise and those specific muscles and joints get warmed up, you may discover that you can increase your range of motion. You may also find that a larger range of motion may get uncomfortable as you complete more reps and may choose to lessen it for now.

4. Avoid fatigue by figuring out how much and how often you need to rest. I've had some beginners need a breather between individual exercises whereas others were able to limit their rest periods to between rounds. It is better to rest and thus be able to work longer than to push through without rest and have your workout end due to fatigue.

Be sure to record all this data in your training log.

You may choose to stick to alternating these circuits two or three times per week for the first four to six weeks of your new training experience. If you can complete an entire circuit with no rest at all, it is time to increase the difficulty by adding resistance or additional exercises. In Chapter Eight, I will teach you how to build workouts including more exercises.

There is an exhaustive list of exercises that build on these basic movements in Appendix A. It is important that you master these six movements and keep them in regular rotation for good joint health.

As you will see, it is possible to do these circuits in as little as twenty minutes, so they should easily fit into your schedule at home or at the office.

* * *

The ultimate goal of learning and practicing these movements is to use them in your everyday activities. You will squat in and out of your chair. You will deadlift heavy objects off the ground. You will maintain good spinal posture and core stability when pushing objects away from yourself, pulling them toward yourself, rotating your shoulders, and any other movement you engage in throughout your day. Your muscles will be active, your posture will be stable, and you will move with strength and purpose.

CHAPTER 7

POWER TRAINING AND WEIGHTED CARRIES

———

One of my good friends and colleagues Mike McKenna is a USA Weightlifting National coach who owns a training facility in Highland Park, New Jersey. Like many coaches of high-level athletes, he supplements his income by training everyday folks who just want to get stronger and live a better life. Since explosive barbell lifts are his passion, pretty much everyone who comes into his gym, regardless of age or ability, has some sort of power movement as part of their training plan.

What do I mean by power movements?

Power movements can be described as moving the body explosively in a coordinated fashion to deliver a blow, lift a weight, or throw an object. Sprinting, jumping, pitching a baseball, throwing a punch, swinging a bat, and swinging an axe are all power movements.

For Mike, this technique means that although his younger and more able clients will be snatching and cleaning barbells, everyone else is going to be participating by swinging kettle-bells, throwing medicine balls, and jumping as part of their workouts. For them to participate safely in power training, Mike has all his clients build their strength foundation first with the traditional exercises as I've outlined in Chapter Six, and when they are ready, he adds some appropriate power movements to the mix.

One of the stories Mike has told me over the years is of a group of older women, in their sixties and seventies, who would come train with him a few times a week. At the beginning of their workout, he would take them outside, put them on two sides of the yard out back, and have them throw big inflatable balls back and forth to one another. It was fun, it got them outside, it raised their heart rates, but most impor-tantly, it had them repeating a movement that required them to push through their legs, stabilize their cores, and extend their arms and shoulders explosively. For these ladies it was just a fun way to warm up; nevertheless, the actual benefits were far greater.

Power movements in general utilize your entire body to deliver a tremendous amount of force in an extremely short amount of time. As with strength training, power training greatly improves coordination. Since these movements are performed rapidly, they are more metabolically taxing than slower strength exercises, so performing them repeatedly can also be a great conditioning tool. Most importantly, these exercises tend to be full body movements, meaning they utilize the muscles of the upper body, lower body, and core.

As I stated in Chapter Six, we are not made of individually acting muscle segments. Our bodies are continuous chains of muscle groups that work in synchrony, so whenever we can practice movements that utilize those chains as a whole, we are going to improve our body's ability to function.

Power movements are one kind of full-body movement, but many other exercises can provide similar benefits. The truth is most of our movements in life are full-body. Bending over to pick up a laundry basket and carry it to the washing machine, unloading and carrying bags of mulch or groceries from the back of the car, picking up and carrying a baby, the list goes on and on.

When we discussed the evolutionary advantages of walking in Chapter Four, I made mention of one of the great advantages of walking on two legs: *being able to walk and carry things at the same time.* I would like to introduce probably one of the greatest and easiest full body movements you can add to your training program: weighted carries. Carrying a heavy object—whether it be a bag of mulch, a bag of sand, or a pair of weights—requires a lot of effort, especially from your core.

Power movements and weighted carries can play a number of roles in your workouts. For most general fitness goals, they can become part of your strength circuit or be used as a conditioning tool at the end of a workout. Of course, as stated above, if you keep them light, they can also be a fun way to warm up your body and get ready for your workout.

KETTLEBELL SWINGS

I love kettlebells. I used to teach a strength and conditioning class that was solely based on kettlebell movements. It was great because you only used one implement, the kettlebell, for the class, and I would instruct my attendees through a series of short circuits that included squats, lunges, presses, and of course, the kettlebell swing.

The kettlebell swing is a great full-body exercise. It hits your hips, your core, your upper back, and your shoulders. You can perform it standing in place, which greatly reduces your likelihood of tripping over your own feet (this is very important to me). It can be a stand-alone workout if you're short on time and don't mind swinging a kettlebell off and on for ten minutes.

The kettlebell swing can seem confusing to understand when you first see one in motion, but once you understand the mechanics of it, it makes a lot more sense. What I mean by that is since you are holding on to the kettlebell with your hands, may people mistakenly think you are primarily swinging it with your arms. In reality, the primary driver of the kettlebell swing is your hips.

In figure 7.1a, Patrick is at the bottom of his kettlebell swing. Make a note of his straight back posture. This is very similar to the posture you would use on a squat or a deadlift. The kettlebell has swung down between his legs, and he has squatted down to let his arms follow through.

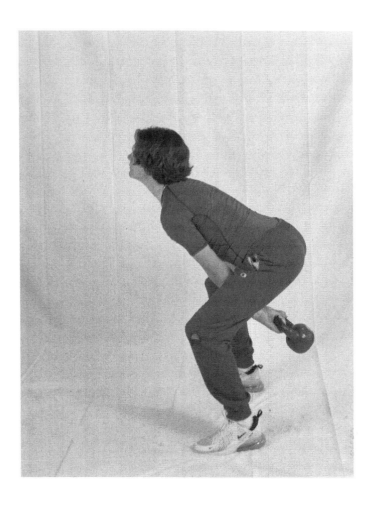

Figure 7.1a: Kettlebell Swing Bottom

At this point of the swing, his forearms are in contact with his thighs, and he is about to powerfully straighten his legs and hips to reverse the motion of the kettlebell so that it swings forward. His hips and legs will create momentum, and the bell will swing up past his hips, as in figure 7.1b.

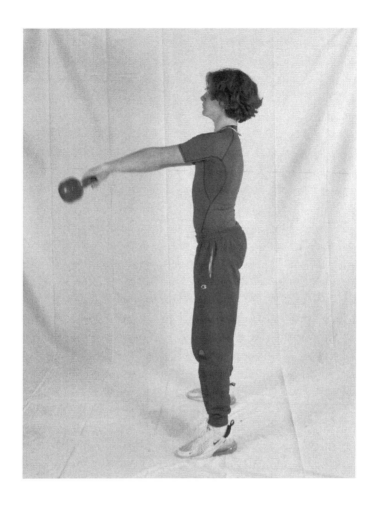

Figure 7.1b: Kettlebell Swing Middle

It is important to note that through the duration of the swing, Patrick's upper back is also actively engaged to maintain that straight-back, open-chest posture. As the bell swings past his hips, his hips are fully extended, and he will begin to assist its rise by actively raising his arms and shoulders until they are about eye-level before he lets it drop back down. Figure 7.1c shows the top position of the kettlebell.

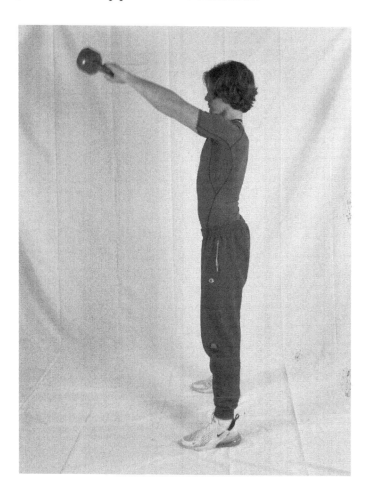

Figure 7.1c: Kettlebell Swing Top

Once you get the hang of kettlebell swings, you can put them in any number of places in your workout. You can use them as a stand-alone exercise in the beginning of your workout, you can include them in your strength circuit to keep your heart rate up and provide some full body stimulus, or you can use them as a conditioning tool at the end of your workout. If I'm having a day where I want to do "something" but just don't have the time or feel motivated for a full workout, I'll just do kettlebell swings. Maybe I'll do five to eight sets of fifteen swings, or maybe I'll just aim to do one hundred total in however many sets it takes to get me there.

You don't necessarily need a kettlebell to do swings. You can use a single dumbbell or even a milk jug full of sand. If you want to purchase a kettlebell to use for swings, I recommend starting with one that is ten to fifteen pounds for women and twenty to twenty-five pounds for men. If you can, try a few different sizes out before purchasing. I have kettlebells that go from five pounds to sixty-five pounds, but I consistently use my fifteen and twenty pound bells the most.

MEDICINE BALL THROWS

Well, I must admit, I also love medicine balls. It might be because I like throwing things, but I love how versatile they are, and I also love that you can use them with a partner. A favorite mini-circuit of mine is to have clients alternate between medicine ball slams and Russian twists. A medicine ball slam is basically a violent standing abdominal crunch that also works the shoulders and upper back. The Russian twist, as you know from Chapter Six, is a rotational movement. Together, they target the core, upper back, and shoulders.

MEDICINE BALL SLAMS

As I described above, a medicine ball slam is a violent standing crunch in which you basically throw the medicine ball at the ground with great force. It is pretty much the opposite movement of the kettlebell swing above. These exercises are actually fun to do back and forth with a partner as well, you just have to pay attention so that you not only catch the ball your partner throws, but so you don't get hit by it either.

In figure 7.2a, Patrick is preparing to throw the ball by swinging it over and behind his head. You don't have to swing it back as far as Patrick has it. It's perfectly fine to raise it up over your head or even in front. The main goal is that you give yourself plenty of a wind up to reverse the movement and slam it into the ground which is exactly what Patrick is doing in figure 7.2b. The difference between these two photos is Patrick's hip position. Before he initiates the slam, his hips are straight. As he starts to bring the ball down, his hips start to flex. No matter where you start your throw, you want your hips to be fully extended, i.e., straight, before you start your slam.

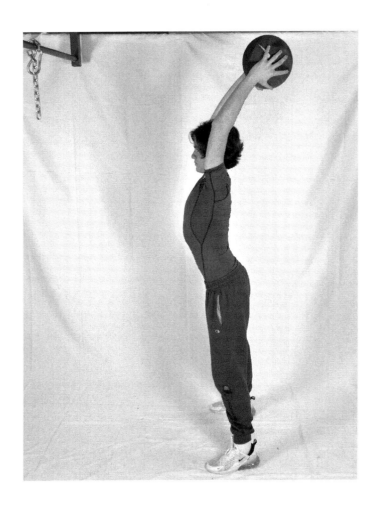

Figure 7.2a: Medicine Ball Slam Beginning

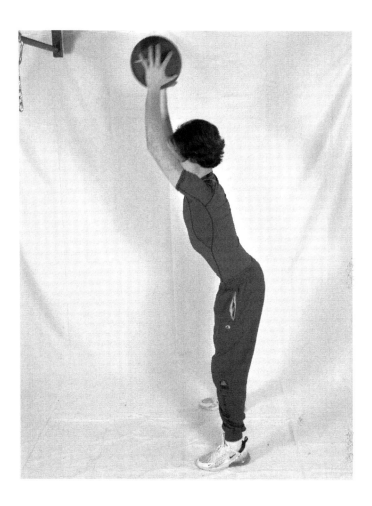

Figure 7.2b: Medicine Ball Slam Middle

In figure 7.2c, Patrick has completed the slam, and the ball has hit the ground and bounced back up. Once you get into a rhythm with these slams, you can easily catch the ball and continue with your repetitions. In figure 7.2d, Francis and Shani are slamming the medicine ball back and forth with it bouncing between them.

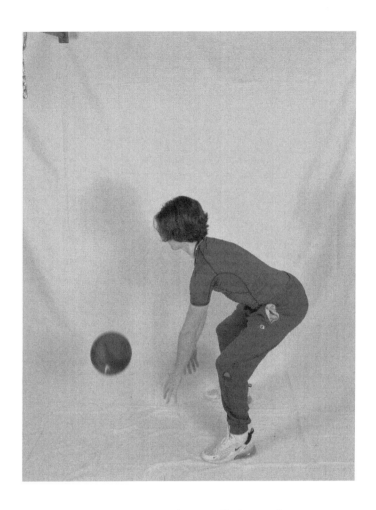

Figure 7.2c: Medicine Ball Slam End

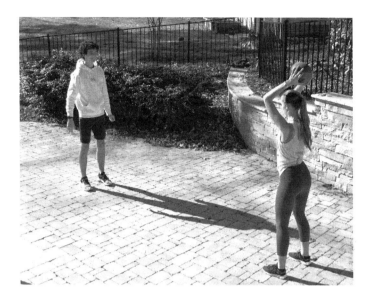

Figure 7.2d: Medicine Ball Slam with Partner

MEDICINE BALL SIDE THROW

Side throws are basically a standing Russian twist with a more violent ending in which you let go of the ball. For this reason, it's a good idea to have either a wall to throw it into or a partner to catch it. When we perform a standing Russian twist, we have to decelerate the weight as we approach the opposite side, or else we risk hurting ourselves. When we can let go of the weight, we can continue to accelerate all the way through, similarly to how we would swing a baseball bat or a golf club.

To perform a side throw, stand sideways to a wall or your partner (if you have a partner, don't stand too close, it can get dangerous). Rotate your upper body and the ball away from the direction you are going to throw, as in figure 7.3, and then quickly reverse your movement. Release the ball as you turn toward the wall or your partner. When I do side throws against a wall, I like to stand far enough back that it bounces before it hits the wall, so I have some time to react and catch it. As with slams, you can get into a rhythm where you can easily complete multiple repetitions without stopping.

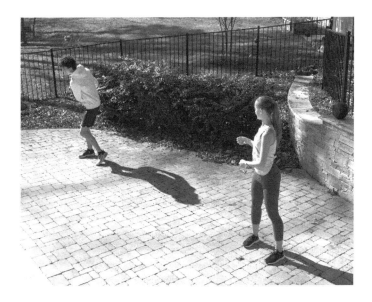

Figure 7.3: med ball side throw

MEDICINE BALL PUSH PRESS THROW

A push press is a regular overhead press that is assisted with some leg drive. You bend your hips and knees slightly at the beginning of the lift and then forcefully extend them as you push the weights overhead. A push press throw is basically an overhead throw that uses the same mechanics as a push press, only you get to let go of the ball.

This exercise can be done in three ways. You can throw the ball into a wall and have it bounce back to you, you can throw it freely and pick it up once it lands, or you can throw it back and forth with a partner. Unless you are throwing it at a wall, this particular exercise lends itself to using a slam ball for a couple of reasons. A slam ball is usually filled with sand and doesn't bounce so it won't get away from you. Slam balls are also a lot heavier than regular medicine balls so you can exert more force.

In the first figures 7.4a and 7.4b, Shani is throwing a regular medicine ball at a wall. She holds the ball in front of her chest, and as with the kettlebell swing, she bends her knees and hips and quickly reverses as she pushes the ball overhead. Her hips and legs deliver a lot more power than her arms, so this tends to be more of a lower body and core exercise, although it does benefit the arms and shoulders as well.

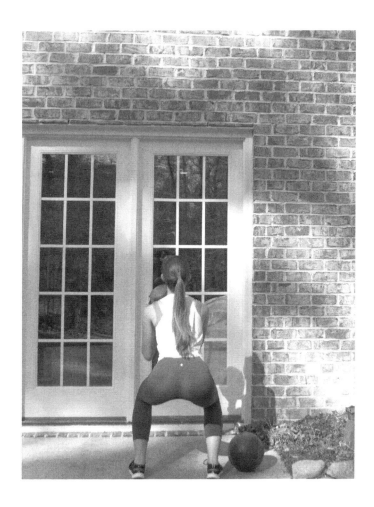

Figure 7.4a: Medicine Ball Push Press Throw Beginning

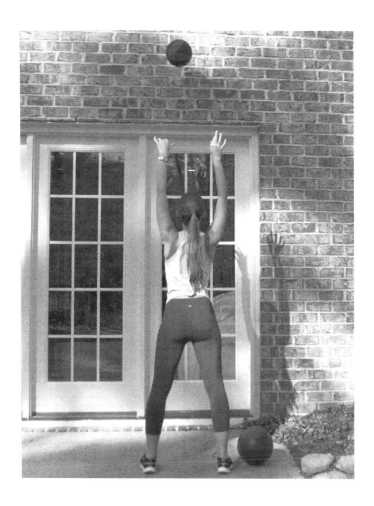

Figure 7.4b: Medicine Ball Push Press Throw End

In figure 7.4c, Shani is throwing a twenty-pound slam ball as opposed to the four-pound medicine ball she is using in the first two photos. The reason heavier weights are appropriate with this throw is because this throw relies on the larger muscles of the shoulders and a straight line of force from the chest rather than the more full-range-of-motion movements required by the slams and side throws.

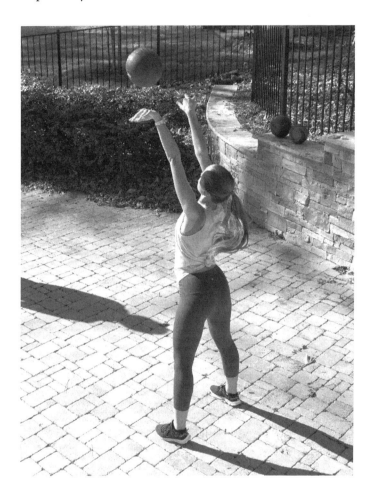

Figure 7.4c: Slam Ball Push Press Throw

Medicine balls are a great tool, but you don't need a lot of weight for an effective workout. For most women, four to six pounds is plenty of weight. I might increase that to six to eight pounds for men, but not much more. Of course, you can always start with an unweighted ball and throw it however you like. The dynamic nature of medicine ball movements allows for free movement of the hips and shoulders, and lighter weights allow for far more versatility.

JUMPS

Jumping is one of those things we all did as a kid without even thinking about it. I will fully admit that the idea of jumping at almost fifty years old fills me with a little trepidation. However, jumping is a great movement. In fact, jumping has been shown to safely improve strength, balance, ankle flexibility, and bone density in older adults up to seventy-nine years old.[117]

Jumping can take on a number of forms and can be as simple as doing jumping jacks or jumping rope. You can even perform small hops in place while holding on to a stationary object to help you balance. These are great exercises to add to your warm-up, since they don't take a lot of time to complete but will still get your heart rate up and all your muscles firing.

BOX JUMPS

The box jump is something that many of you have probably seen due to its popularity in high-intensity fitness workouts. I think box jumps are a great exercise, but they are not something I want to see in the middle of an intense workout. The

---

117 Tomas Vetrovsky et al., "The Efficacy and Safety of Lower-Limb Plyometric Training in Older Adults: A Systematic Review," *Sports Medicine* 49, no. 1 (January 1, 2019): 125–8.

reason is that they require a good bit of coordination. In figure 7.6a, Francis is beginning his box jump by swinging his arms back and beginning to push his hips back and squat down. Note that he is standing about a foot's width back from the box to give himself plenty of room to reach the box height. He is also looking down at the box, so he knows where he wants to land. Always look before you leap!

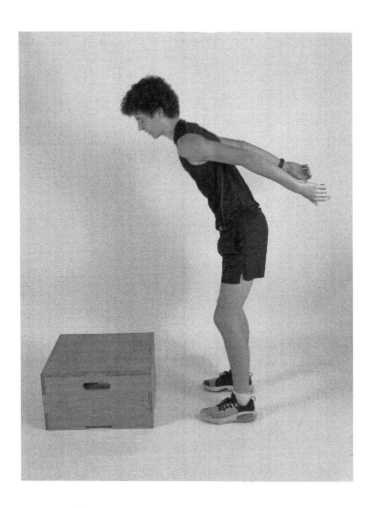

Figure 7.6a: Box Jump Start

He will probably squat down a few more inches before explosively pushing off the ground with his legs and swinging his arms forward and up, as in figure 7.6b. He will land on the box with knees and hips bent, i.e., bent, to absorb the shock of his landing. One of the cues I give trainees new to jumping is, "light as a feather." I want them to land as softly as possible to reduce the amount of force their joints have to absorb. Once he lands, Francis will step down off the box before completing another repetition. Some people will jump up and back down off the box, but I find this quickly leads to joint pain and tendonitis in the knees, hips, and ankles in a lot of people, so I highly recommend you step down and don't jump off the box.

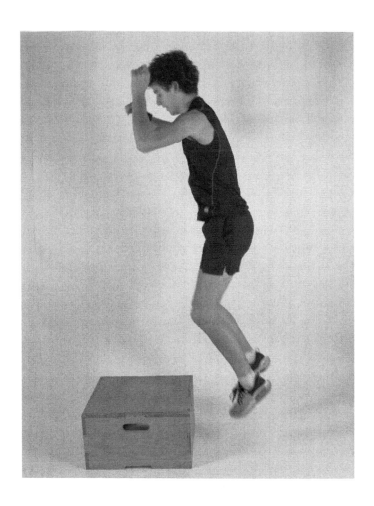

Figure 7.6b: Box Jump Middle

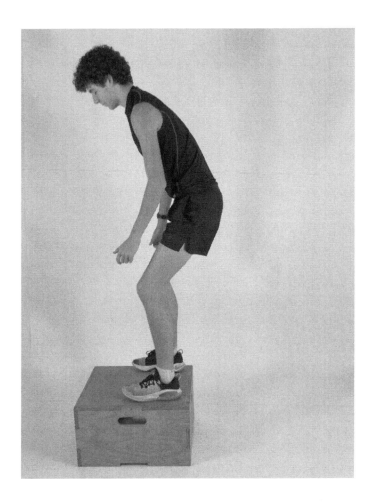

Figure 7.6c: Box Jump Finish

The box Francis is jumping onto is twelve inches high. I have a four-inch aerobic step that I use for some beginner clients as well as an 8 x 18 inch box. Anything higher than eighteen inches isn't really necessary. As boxes get higher and higher, most people aren't actually jumping that high, they are simply pulling their knees up higher and higher to clear the top of the box, and I think that's a bit silly. The average vertical jump height for women is 12–19 inches, and for men, this height is 16–23 inches.[118] Focus on good mechanics and power. Three to five reps at a time is plenty. You can do multiple sets, but give yourself a minute or two of recovery time between each.

SANDBAGS

When I first left the commercial gym I was training in and moved into my basement, I did not have a lot of equipment besides pull-up bars and dumbbells. The bars and squat racks I ordered weren't going to come in for four to six weeks, and I was desperate to find some good training tools. Sandbags were the answer.

I made my sandbags out of army duffle bags and rubber mulch and tied them closed with a zip tie. I had a range of weights from thirty-five pounds to seventy pounds for my larger men. Because sandbags are relatively awkward to handle, they don't have to be particularly heavy to be challenging to be effective.

One of my favorite exercises is the sandbag "clean and shoulder." A clean is a movement where you lift an object by rapidly extending your hips. Any time you have had a child or grocery bag sliding down off your hip and you quickly jumped it back into place, you are performing a version of a clean. The clean is also a barbell movement in which you

---

118 Jay, "Average Vertical Jump: Norms and Scores," *Jumping Universe* (blog), August 18, 2020.

explosively move the bar from your knees to your shoulders. It is part of the "clean and jerk," an event in the sport of Olympic weightlifting.

In figure 7.9a, Laura starts out with the sandbag between her feet. She grasps it firmly in both hands and essentially dead-lifts it straight up to the position we see in figure 7.9b. In this figure, her hips are back, and her knees are bent, which sets her up to be able to explosively extend her hips and knees as she pulls the sandbag up over her shoulder, as in figure 7.9c.

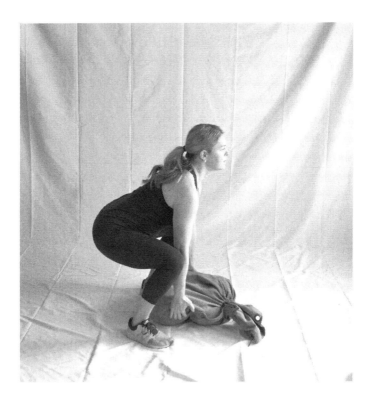

Figure 7.9a: Sandbag Between Feet

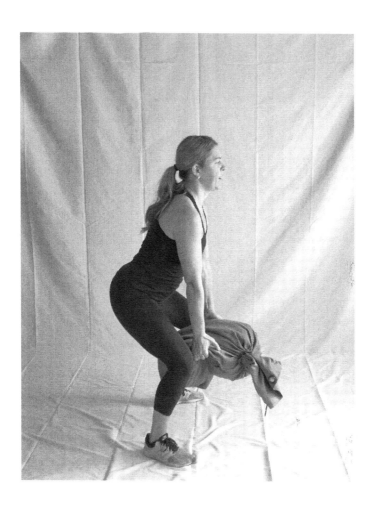

Figure 7.9b: Sandbag Pick

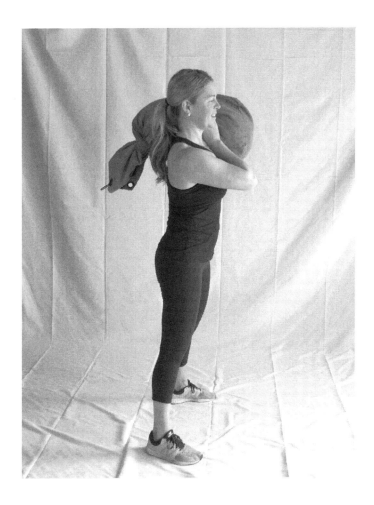

Figure 7.9c: Sandbag Shoulder

She will then drop the bag back onto the floor and then begin again only pulling it to the opposite shoulder. She will continue alternating shoulders until all her reps are complete.

This exercise requires full-body coordination and a lot of core strength. It also requires a lot of oxygen and is, therefore, a great conditioning tool. The shoulders, back, core, hips, and legs are all targeted by this exercise, and it can be a stand-alone workout when you are short on time. For a short conditioning workout, try doing five to ten sets of ten total reps (five each side) with a minute or two of rest between each set.

WEIGHTED CARRIES

Weighted carries are a fantastic exercise and most of us do them on a regular basis without realizing it. Carrying heavy objects is probably one of the best ways to highlight any postural strength issues you may have. When we pick up bags of groceries, bags of mulch, gallons of milk, etc., the weight tends to start pulling us down from the shoulders and tipping us forward. To counteract the weight of our carried objects, we need to pull our shoulders back, lift our chests up, stabilize our core muscles, and let our legs do the work. Carrying heavy objects incorrectly puts unfavorable forces on our joints and can cause injury. Practicing carrying heavy objects correctly, whether in our workouts or in our latest trip to the hardware store, reinforces good movement patterns and postural strength.

In figure 7.10, Patrick is carrying two sixty-pound kettlebells in what is known as a farmer's carry. This not only challenges his postural strength, but also his grip strength. Because he is on uneven ground (grass), he walks with his toes pointed up as he steps forward to avoid tripping. You can use virtually anything in a farmer's carry: kettlebells, dumbbells, buckets of water, hay bales, etc. The idea is simply that it's easier to carry two heavy objects than just one because it helps you keep your balance. With my clients, I will mark off a certain distance (typically fifty feet) for the objects to be carried, and we repeat this distance multiple times. If the carrier needs to put the objects down briefly, they can. You may find that your grip strength fatigues more quickly than anything else.

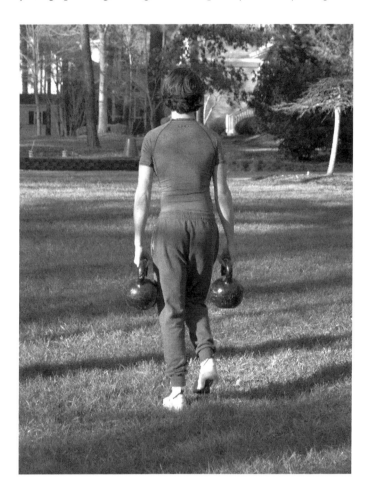

Figure 7.10: Farmer's Carry

You can perform weighted carries with virtually anything and are not limited to just carrying objects in your hands. I will also have clients bear hug or shoulder a sandbag and walk with that as well. These are a great thing to couple with one or two more exercises to do a circuit outside in your yard, your driveway, or a local park. For example, do ten push-ups, carry a sandbag fifty feet, do ten more push-ups and carry it back. Or, have a partner stand thirty to fifty feet away from you. Clean and shoulder your sandbag ten times, carry it to your partner and run back to your starting line. Those things sound easy to do, but I can assure you they are not. You can add some push-ups and squats to the mix if you are feeling particularly energetic, but simple is better.

CHAPTER 8

BUILDING WORKOUTS

———

I am hoping by now that I have convinced you of a couple of things:

1. Walking, and movement in general, is deeply important to our health and wellness and if nothing else, we should be getting up out of our chairs often and moving our bodies as much as possible.
2. Strength training is deeply important to our ability to function pain-free and live an active life.

Now, I would like to convince you that incorporating both of these things into your lifestyle will neither be hard nor time consuming and that your life will be better for it. Easy, right?

Walking to deal with the COVID-19 lockdown of 2020 and the death of my mother was like medicine for my body and mind. After a few months, however, I knew I needed to add some strength training back into my exercise regimen. My knees and back had been bothering me a bit, and before it got worse, I started heading down to my basement a couple times a week to do what I could to mitigate that. My workouts were simple, and I used light weights—nothing more than the basic exercises outlined in Chapter Six, with a few extras such as kettlebell swings, face pulls, and step-ups. This is basic foundational fitness, the fitness that allows you to have an active functional life.

This simple approach works, and it works well. If I want to start competing again, at anything, I have this great foundation to build from; however, I don't need to be in top competitive form to live a good life. In fact, I would argue that constantly being in competition form makes it hard to have time to enjoy a good life, and as I get older, it takes its toll on my body as well.

A friend of mine, Justin Keane, has been running a strength gym centered around group fitness for the past decade in Littleton, Massachusetts, just north of Boston. His training principles, in his own words, mirror my own advice, and I think he says it best:

Our approach is based on these principles:

- *Start with an assessment.*
- *Make low-level cardio (e.g., walking, hiking, riding, etc.) a priority outside of the gym.*
- *Focus on major movement patterns that mirror what we do in life.*
- *Win every workout.*
- *Focus on one small improvement at a time.*
- *Help people develop a relationship with their own fitness from day one, rather than seeing it as something beyond their reach.*

- *Every time we have strayed from these principles in search of something brighter and shinier, it's been a mistake. High-intensity workouts and byzantine eating and training protocols may make for attractive social media, but they rarely make sense for the great majority of folks who are just looking to feel better, move better, and enjoy their lives a little bit more.*
- *Walk. Lift. Keep it simple. And then keep keeping it simple.*
  JUSTIN KEANE, WOODSHED FITNESS

In this chapter, I'm going to teach you how to build your own foundational training program. I'm going to teach you to build workouts, incorporate some aerobic fitness, and make both a regular part of your routine. The most important thing to keep in mind is not to add too much too soon. If we overwhelm ourselves too early, we aren't likely to continue. The most important thing here is that we continue.

HOW TO STRUCTURE A WORKOUT

What exactly is a workout?

It's a good question to ask. Some people think of an exercise class at a fitness facility. Others may think of a weight training session focusing on a specific body part. When I use the term "workout" in this book, I am referring to an exercise session that primarily focuses on strength but may include some other elements such as skill development or conditioning. For most people, two to three workouts per week are adequate to improve strength, especially if they are practicing those skills and postures outside of their workout sessions and are engaging in regular general activity such as walking or gardening.

When building your workouts, it's good to start with two that you alternate between. For many of my beginners, I alternate them between two workouts three times per week. So, Monday they do workout one, Wednesday they do workout two, Friday they do workout one, again, and then on Monday of the following week they start with workout two. If they have to skip a workout, they just start back with the next workout in the sequence. Depending on how many workouts you have, your schedule can look any number of ways:

	2 work-outs	3 work-outs	4 work-outs	2 work-outs	3 work-outs	4 work-outs
Monday	1	1	1	1	1	1
Tuesday				2	2	2
Wednesday	2	2	2			
Thursday						3
Friday	1	3	3	1	3	4
Saturday				2	1	
Sunday						
Monday	2	1	4	1	2	1

The key is to make these sessions as effective and safe as possible. Remember this one thing: **as the body fatigues, coordination decreases.** This concept is very important to remember because it will dictate what elements you include and where you include them in your workouts. Depending on your fitness level, fatigue may be something that becomes an issue early on in your session or isn't really an issue at all. Regardless, we need to think about structuring our workouts in the following way:

1. Warm-up
2. Skill work (optional)
3. Strength circuit
4. Conditioning work (optional)
5. Aerobic training (optional)
6. Stretching (optional-ish)

Warming up: A warm-up gets your blood flowing, your muscles warm, and your neurons firing. Advanced athletes will spend a great deal of time on their warm-ups to be as physically ready as possible for the long work ahead. For most of us, that's not necessary. Move your body, bend and flex all your joints, swing your arms and legs, etc. You can march in place, walk backwards, forwards, and sideways, or do jumping jacks. This should take no more than five minutes.

The warm-up routine I outlined in Chapter Six is a good place to start.

Skill work: This is the time to try out a new exercise or practice one you are having a hard time with. This is learning. If you have a new skill you want to master, just set aside ten minutes or so to practice it without any other distractions. This is a good place to put any stand-alone power work such as medicine ball throws or box jumps.

Pull-ups are a common exercise that some of my clients work on during this portion of the workout. I have them work through five to eight sets of three to five repetitions of either assisted pull-ups with a partner or band, or negatives (this is when you jump or use a step to get into the top position and lower yourself down slowly).* This allows them to work on these when they are still fresh and can rest as much as they want between sets without worrying about doing other exercises.

See Appendix A for more information on pull-ups and pull-up variations.

Strength Circuit: This is the main part of your workout. Typically, three to six exercises performed one after the other in multiple rounds. Typically, ten to fifteen reps per exercise, three to five total rounds, will be ideal for most exercises. For exercises that you find particularly difficult, such as pull-ups, lowering the rep count range to five to ten is acceptable.

Rest between rounds is ideal. If you don't need rest between rounds, your workout might be a little too easy, and you may need to add some weight or complexity.* If you need rest after each exercise, your workout might be a little too difficult. That's okay at first and when adding new exercises, but ideally, being able to steadily work through a single round should be one of your goals.

If you are using a larger number of exercises, you can break this up into two circuits with three to four exercises each. I like doing this when setting up for one circuit would require too much equipment or too many position changes. For example, I can make one circuit of exercises that all utilize a kettlebell (goblet squats, kettlebell swings, step ups with a press) and then make a second circuit that has exercises I do on a mat (push-ups, supermans, medicine ball sit-ups.)

Adding complexity means adding some additional movement to an exercise. For example, if you are performing step-ups onto a box, you can add complexity by adding an overhead press with a medicine ball each time you step up onto the box. You can find a comprehensive list of additional exercises and instruction in Appendix B.

Conditioning Work: This is where we can play a little bit and get our heart rates up. Remember how Seiler proposed that only 20 percent of training should go into the yellow or red zone? This is that zone. Remember that this is an enhancement to your regular training and should not take over as the main mode of training. Training at higher intensities all the time limits progress and increases your risk of injury, so we keep these short and "fun." (That depends on your definition of fun.)

Some power movements and weighted carries are a great choice here, although you could also do some interval training with some running, rowing, or jumping rope (or fake jumping rope if you have a hard time not tripping over the rope like I do.) You can use a single exercise or perform a circuit of two to three exercises. The difference between these exercises and your strength circuit is that these are typically much shorter (five to eight minutes), have shorter rest periods, and do induce fatigue.

You should feel remarkably tired when you are done with your conditioning work. The benefits of these little "finisher" sessions are that you can focus on doing work with more resistance and good form during your strength session, and then use these to get your heart rate up and finish the session a little sweaty and tired.

You can use several formats for these finishers. My favorite is EMOM, or "Every Minute On the Minute." For this type of finisher, you pick one exercise such as swinging a kettlebell, jumping rope, or shouldering a sandbag. Every minute, you perform a certain number of reps with the idea of continuously working for fifteen to forty-five seconds. You have the remainder of the minute to rest before starting over again. The decreased recovery time is much more taxing than you may think, and you will find yourself very tired, very quickly.

Another format you can use is micro-intervals. If you've ever heard of the Tabata protocol, where you work for twenty seconds and rest for ten, this is an example of a micro-interval. All this means is that your total work and rest periods are under a minute. EMOM is a form of a micro-interval, but if you'd rather have a set work time, this format is more precise. When you are just starting out with this technique, it's better to have a shorter work period and longer rest period. As you improve your conditioning, you can shorten the rest period and take a longer work period.

Examples of Micro-intervals

Work	Rest
15 s	45 s
30 s	30 s
45 s	15 s
1 m	30 s
30 s	15 s
1 m	1 m

Important to note, these short conditioning workouts are very effective at boosting your overall conditioning, however, they are *not* a substitute for longer-duration, lower-intensity aerobic training. I can't tell you how many clients I have trained who came from gyms where this was all the "cardio" they would do, and no matter how strong they were, they lacked the stamina and endurance to get through my weight training sessions. They are powerful, so use them sparingly. Once or twice a week is enough to yield considerable benefits from them.

Aerobic Training: I think it's a great idea to finish a workout with a twenty-minute walk, jog, or row. It helps relax any tight muscles and stimulates blood flow, which helps with recovery. Obviously, aerobic training can be a workout all by itself, and there are some different ways you can structure these workouts as well by utilizing some interval training concepts. As we discussed in Chapter One, thirty to forty-five minutes of aerobic training a day is plenty, and you don't have to do it all at once. Two twenty-minute sessions or even three ten-minute sessions are equally beneficial.

For standalone daily aerobic training, weight bearing exercise such as walking, dancing, or running are great. Biking, rowing, and swimming are also good. Just go out and enjoy yourself!

If you are looking to increase the speed or distance that you cover when doing your aerobic training, incorporating the concept of interval training into your workouts is an easy way to do that. The most basic kind of interval training is fartlek training. Fartlek is Swedish for "speed play," and although the original term applied to running, it can be used with all kinds of endurance modes. The basic idea is to go at a slightly challenging pace until you start to fatigue or get out of breath. You then drop to a slower pace to recover and continue with this rhythm until you can proceed at a challenging pace again.

Most of our volume endurance training, that 80 percent green zone training that Seiler speaks about, should be done at a pace where we are not out of breath and could hold a conversation if necessary. This could simply mean jogging for a few minutes and then walking to recover. Ideally, you will be able to push the pace of the more challenging intervals over time and/or reduce the amount of time in recovery. Ultimately, you will be able to sustain the "challenging" pace over longer periods of time until it's your new "easy" pace.

I used this approach a great deal with my cross-country runners. The sixth graders new to running would get pretty overwhelmed at the beginning of the season. The problem was that they would start out running fast and quickly run out of breath. Then, of course, they would be tired and feel awful and want to walk the remainder of the distance. There was usually a lot of whining as I would try to encourage these tired little people to finish their workout.

Instead of arguing with them, I would pick a landmark a relatively short distance ahead, maybe a street sign or a mailbox, and I'd have them run to that landmark and then walk, hopefully before they started to feel worn out. Once they were able to talk again (keeping sixth graders from talking to their friends is almost impossible), I'd pick another landmark and have them run to that. Without realizing it, they typically ran twice the distance they would if left to their own devices.

Another way to use interval training is by using a timer. I have a treadmill in my basement, and whenever I decide to get back in running shape, I start off by warming up and then alternating a jogging and walking pace every two minutes. I start off doing this for twenty-five minutes and gradually work up to forty-five minutes. Essentially, I increase my jogging time from twelve minutes to twenty-two minutes. From there, I lengthen the jogging intervals and shorten the walking intervals, maybe three minutes on, one minute off, until I can run straight through without stopping.

Stretching: Above, I say this is optional-ish. What I mean by that is that if you have some noticeably tight muscles or pain, you really should stretch them out before ending your session. It won't take more than five minutes and can make a big difference in your comfort level and mobility over time. However, the good thing about stretching is that it can be done at any time of the day. So, you don't necessarily have to stretch during your workout, but I would highly recommend you spend some time stretching at some point throughout your day. A trainer colleague of mine, Tom Furman, recommends stretching several times a day to counter the long hours spent sitting at a desk or driving. He feels that taking a minute or two a couple of times a day to stretch your hips and back is more effective for the long term than limiting your stretching only to workout sessions.

The easiest way to do this is to simply stand up, raise up your arms to your sides, push your hips forward and your head and chest up, lean back a little, and pull your arms back. This stretches your hip flexors and your chest muscles, which tend to tighten when sitting and pull you into a slouched posture.

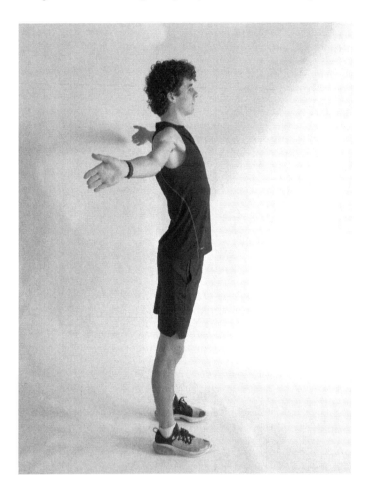

Figure 8.1: Standing Stretch

You can identify some specific stretches from Chapter Eight or use the following stretching routine below. This is the stretching routine I do with my cross-country runners and young athletes after a training session. Try to hold each stretch for ten to thirty seconds and repeat each one three to five times with a few seconds rest between attempts.

Cool Down Stretches

	Body Part	Instructions
Modified Uttanasana (This Is a Yoga Stretch)	Spine and Hamstrings	Bend over while bending your knees and try to reach your toes. Hold on to whatever you are able to reach (toes, shoelaces, ankles, etc.) Take a deep breath, and as you let it out, straighten your knees without releasing your hands. Count to ten and bend your knees again to release the tension.
Double Leg Stretch Forward	Hips and Legs	Sit on the floor with your legs splayed out to the sides. Reach forward as far as you can with both arms and hold the position.
Double Leg Stretch Side	Hips and Legs	Maintaining the same position as above, alternate stretching both hands toward one foot.
Single Seg Stretch	Hips and Hamstrings	In the position above, tuck one foot in to the middle and reach for the opposite foot.
Lying Hamstring Stretch	Hamstring	Laying on your back, alternate pulling one knee to your chest at a time.
Lower Back Rotation Stretch	Hips and Low Back	Pull one knee to your chest and rotate your hips to the opposite side of the knee such that your knee touches or approaches the floor. Keep your upper back flat on the floor.
Piriformis* Stretch 1	Hips and Low Back	While on your back, lie flat. Pull one knee up and rotate your ankle inward so that your ankle now sits just above the opposite knee. Grab the thigh of the opposite knee and pull toward yourself.

	Body Part	Instructions
Piriformis* Stretch 2	Hips and Back	Sit up with your legs out straight. Pick up one leg and cross it over the other with your knee up. Take your elbow opposite that knee and place it on the outside of the knee and push with your elbow to rotate your torso toward that side.
Shoulder Stretch	Shoulders and Upper Back	You can do this standing or seated. Pull your arm laterally across your chest and press your upper arm into your upper chest.
Triceps Stretch	Triceps and Chest	You can do this standing or seated. Point your elbow straight up. Reach around your head with your other arm and pull your arm backward from the elbow. You can also do this by leaning into a wall with your arm up.

The piriformis is a muscle deep in your pelvis that can get irritated from too much activity or sitting. It can cause discomfort in the legs as well as sciatica.[119]

---

119 Harvard Health Publishing, "Ask Dr. Rob about Piriformis Syndrome," *Harvard Health.*

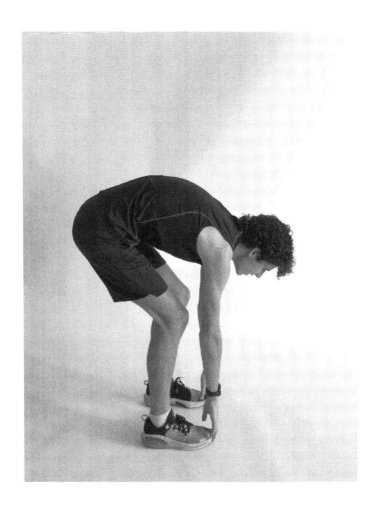

Figure 8.2a: Modified Uttanasana Relaxed

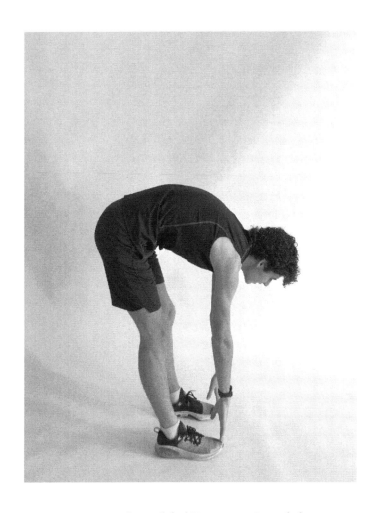

Figure 8.2b: Modified Uttanasana Extended

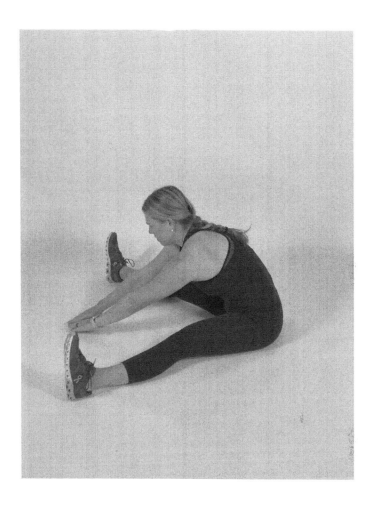

Figure 8.3: Double Leg Stretch Forward

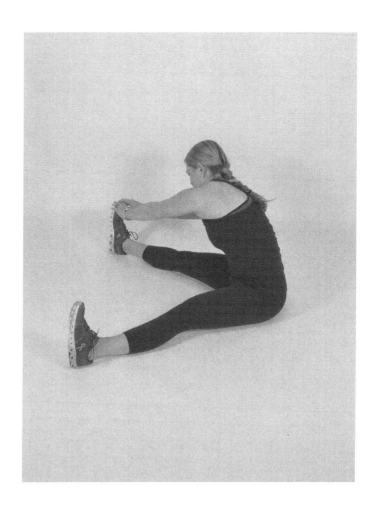

Figure 8.4: Double Leg Stretch Side

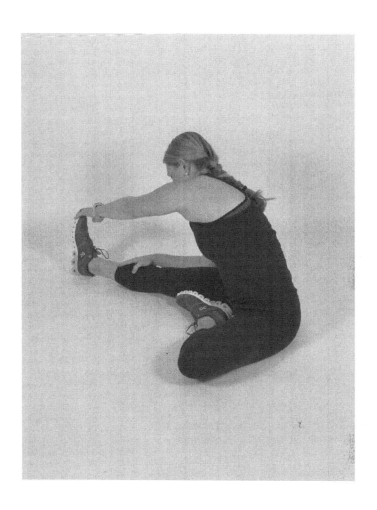

Figure 8.5: Single Leg Stretch

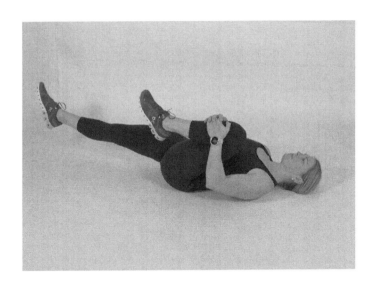

Figure 8.6: Lying Hamstring Stretch

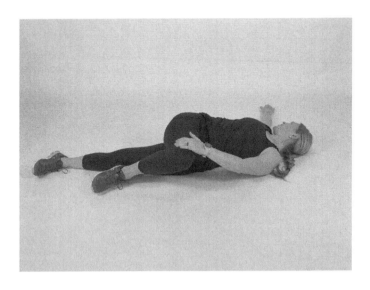

Figure 8.7: Lower Back Rotation Stretch

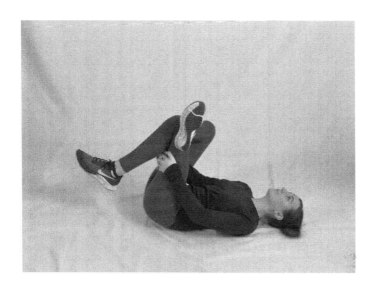

Figure 8.8: Piriformis Stretch 1

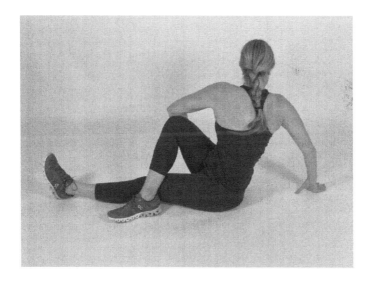

Figure 8.9: Piriformis Stretch 2

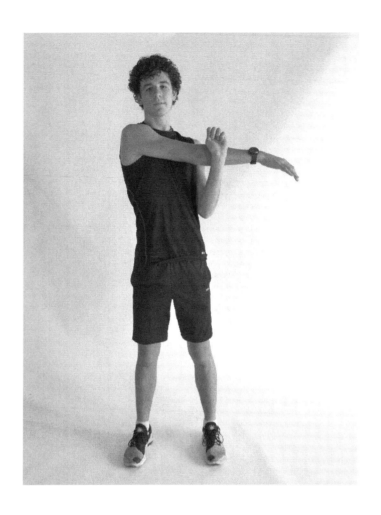

Figure 8.10: Shoulder Stretch

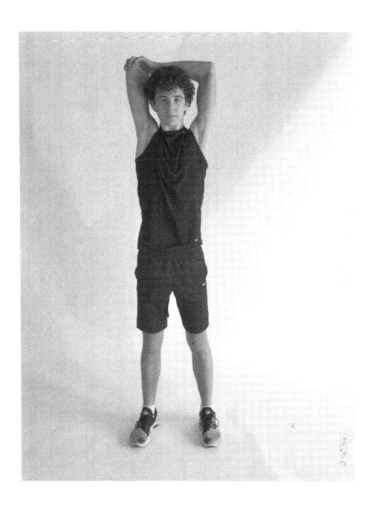

Figure 8.11: Triceps Stretch

At least ten different stretches exist for every muscle in the body. Please do not feel limited by this list. You can easily find stretches that may be more suitable for you on YouTube and countless internet sites. In Appendix A, you will find more specific stretches for each area of the body as well as instructions on how to use foam rolling to help with problem areas.

The most important thing to remember here is that you do not need all seven of these elements in your workout sessions. In fact, the most basic workout form utilizes just one and four, warm-up and a strength circuit. Done. At most, I would add two more elements, for example skill work and cardio, conditioning and stretching, or maybe just power movements and stretching. No matter what you choose to include, don't forget to win the workout!

Eventually, you will be very comfortable designing your own workouts. To get you started, I have described some basic workouts and progressions you can use. Additional exercises are listed in Appendix B. Remember to practice new exercises as skill development before adding them to your workouts.

Workouts Set One: Basic Strength

	Workout 1	Workout 2	Workout 3
	Warm-up	Warm-up	Warm-up
Strength	Circuit of Goblet Squats, push-ups, step-ups, and body rows	Circuit of deadlifts, overhead press, core rotation, face pulls	Circuit of alternating reverse lunges, supermans, plank hold, and lying leg raises
Aerobic	Finish with 20 minute walk or stretching		

Workout Set Two: Power and Strength

	Workout 1	Workout 2	Workout 3
	Warm-up	Warm-up	Warm-up
Power/Skill	Med ball push press throw. 5 sets of 10-15	Box jumps, 5 sets of 5	kettlebell swings, 3-5 sets of 15-25
Strength	Circuit of goblet squats, push-ups, step-ups with overhead press, and core rotation	Circuit of deadlifts, curl and press, assisted pull-ups or rows, and triceps press.	Circuit of walking lunges, wood chops, leg raises, and good mornings.
Aerobic	Optional: Finish with 20 minute walk		

Workout Set 3: Strength and Conditioning

	Workout 1	Workout 2	Workout 3
	Warm-up	Warm-up	Warm-up
Strength	Circuit of goblet squats, push-ups, step-ups, body rows, and core rotation	Circuit of deadlifts, overhead press, bent over rows. Finish with three rounds of shoulder complex, ten reps each exercise.	Circuit of split squats, supermans, plank hold, and lying leg raises
Conditioning	Kettlebell swings, ten to fifteen reps EMOM, five to ten minutes	Medicine ball slams and Russian twists, three to five sets of ten	Sandbag pick up and drop, alternating shoulders, three to five reps each side EMOM for five to eight minutes
	Stretch	Stretch	Stretch

* It is a good idea when using finishers to stretch out the hips and back, especially after the workout. The more intense work will have a tendency to result in some increased muscle soreness and tightness, so addressing it up front is a good idea.

* * *

It doesn't take much to improve how our bodies function with balanced strength training. The biggest mistake I see in the general population when it comes to fitness is thinking that workouts have to be overly complex, long, or intense to make a difference. They don't. You just have to do them with some regularity to see results. Patience and consistency will serve you far better in developing a significant and permanent change in your health and lifestyle. This is where we start. Give yourself some time to build your foundation and from there you can build whatever you like.

CHAPTER 9

STAYING MOTIVATED

It may surprise you to learn that I'm not the most motivated person in the world. If I'm being completely honest with you, I'd prefer to be sitting on my couch watching reruns of *Law and Order* over running a mile any day. Things weren't always this way. When I was younger, I loved getting outside to play sports and ride my bike. Heck, I was even known to go on an exercise binge every now and again when I realized my metabolism wasn't keeping up with my love of pie. However, for the most part, I didn't really enjoy exercising or dieting.

When my babies were small, my husband worked nights in the hospital emergency room, so I joined the local Y because they had a gym and childcare. That meant my kids were watched by responsible adults (who were not me) for two hours while I got some exercise, and more importantly, a shower. If you have three kids under the age of four, a shower by yourself is probably the only thing you deeply care about other than sleep. A kid-free two hours with a shower thrown in was excellent exercise bribery for the time being.

As I got older, and busier, the need for a regular exercise routine became more and more apparent. As I talked about in Chapter One, when you don't regularly maintain that base of fitness as you age, things can start to fall apart rather rapidly. You young folks won't understand this until your mid-thirties. When done poorly, exercise can make small aches and pains so much worse. Regular exercise is also tremendously helpful for your mental health and relieving the stresses of everyday life.[120]

Once I completed my fitness trainer certification, I started training clients at a local CrossFit gym. I would often join in with the gym members after my training sessions to complete the daily workout that occurred during the session after mine. I would leave the gym feeling hungry, exhausted, and accomplished.

Eventually, I developed a craving for some autonomy with the workouts I was coaching. I knew that there were a number of clients who both wanted and needed a more personalized approach to their training, and I wanted the independence that came with having my own workout space. When I acquired all the equipment I needed, I quit my other gym memberships and set up the perfect gym for myself and my clients in my basement.

And then I stopped working out.

---

120 Andrea Camaz Deslandes, "Exercise and Mental Health: What Did We Learn in the Last 20 Years?" *Frontiers in Psychiatry* 5 (2014): 66.

I trained clients for a few months in my home basement gym without doing much of anything myself. I was tired, bored, and lonely. I had lost all motivation. I started to wonder if I actually ever liked working out or if I just craved the camaraderie, attention, and social aspect of it all. This is extrinsic motivation, the motivation based on the expectation of others, and not the best one for a lifetime commitment to fitness. In fact, it has been shown that extrinsic rewards can actually undermine the intrinsic rewards of training.[121]

Let me provide a little more explanation here on these terms. Motivation is most commonly divided into two general types, extrinsic and intrinsic.

Extrinsic motivation can be described as external factors such as how we feel others perceive us. This includes image, acceptance, social recognition, or attractiveness. Praise and rewards, or avoidance of criticism and punishment are other forms of extrinsic motivation.[122] Extrinsic motivation is often the motivation behind starting an exercise program, i.e., wanting a beach body or doing it because your doctor told you to do so.

---

121 Kou Murayama et al., "Neural Basis of the Undermining Effect of Monetary Reward on Intrinsic Motivation," *Proceedings of the National Academy of Sciences* 107, no. 49 (December 7, 2010): 20914–5.

122 Pedro J Teixeira et al., "Exercise, Physical Activity, and Self-Determination Theory: A Systematic Review," *The International Journal of Behavioral Nutrition and Physical Activity* 9:78 (June 22, 2012).; Kylie Wilson and Darren Brookfield, "Effect of Goal Setting on Motivation and Adherence in a Six-Week Exercise Program," *International Journal of Sport and Exercise Psychology* 7, no. 1 (January 1, 2009): 90.

Unfortunately, this does not typically lead to long-term adherence. This is the phenomenon behind the gyms being crowded every year after the holidays and mostly emptying out by June. Everyone wants to lose those extra pounds of holiday cheer and be in shape by summer; however, when the weight doesn't come off immediately and they don't understand the necessity of their exercise routine outside of potential weight loss, they tend to give up.

Intrinsic motivation is focused on the internal factors such as enjoyment of the activity. It also includes feelings of competence and confidence in their abilities to perform the activity as well as autonomy. Autonomy is the concept of taking charge of your own fitness journey, having confidence in your choices, and understanding the utility of the activities you engage in. Autonomy is, perhaps, one of the most powerful motivators for getting people engaged and staying engaged in their own health and wellness.[123]

Although I had been enjoying the intrinsic rewards of learning new training methods and developing competence for myself, the competitive environment of my commercial gym eroded those rewards. I had become focused on the extrinsic rewards of being one of the better athletes in the gym. Back at home, with no one to give me that recognition, working out by myself felt a little pointless.

I enjoyed coaching others, but being a slight introvert, I was too mentally tired after my coaching sessions to motivate

---

123 Teixeira et al., "Exercise, Physical Activity, and Self-Determination Theory: A Systematic Review."

myself to train alone. After a long coaching session, all I wanted to do was lie on the couch with my kids. After all, who doesn't want to spend time with short irrational people who think you are the coolest human who ever existed. Lying on the couch isn't all that unpleasant either.

My lack of motivation and interest in training was not unique. Many fitness programs have a high dropout rate and up to 50 percent of individuals drop out after only three to six months of participation.[124] While we may be evolutionarily hardwired to avoid exercise at all costs, we can work around our evolutionary hard wiring in a number of ways, and it is important to understand how to utilize different types of motivation to keep ourselves on task.[125]

I clearly enjoyed training with others, but I have found that goal setting has been the most effective method for getting me in the gym training. I have found over the years that the goals I enjoy the most are entering a community event or competition. Enjoyment is a key term here because one of the strongest motivators for most people is enjoyment of their activity. Remember that human beings require a certain amount of play in their everyday life. If they can combine that with exercise, they will not only enjoy their workouts, but they will also tend to work harder and more effectively. Depending on your definition of fun, there are many fun competitions out there for the general population

---

124 Wilson and Brookfield, "Effect of Goal Setting on Motivation and Adherence in a Six-Week Exercise Program,": 89.

125 Harold H. Lee, Jessica A. Emerson, and David M. Williams, "The Exercise–Affect–Adherence Pathway: An Evolutionary Perspective," *Frontiers in Psychology* 7:1285 (2016).

to participate in. My first experience with this was the Warrior Dash.

COMPETITION AS MOTIVATION

One afternoon, as I was lying on the couch lamenting my newfound laziness, I came across a YouTube video for a new kind of race called the Warrior Dash. It showed happy, muddy people walking, running, and crawling through mud and climbing over a variety of obstacles. I remember this sense of longing coming over me. I missed being in shape, I missed playing in the mud (okay, that was a much longer time ago, but I still missed it), and I wanted to be with all these happy muddy people who seemed to be having the time of their lives.

The thing that really drew me in was that all these people looked "normal." The lean athletic types I expected to see were surrounded by a large number of people of all ages and body types. Some were running, some were walking, and they were all having fun. You get a furry Viking helmet just for signing up, so I was all in. I wasn't running at all at that time, so I got really excited about coming up with a plan to rebuild that running base as well as the other skills this race would demand.

Over the next couple of weeks, I managed to talk a few of my friends and clients into training with me. Training for this goal would not be about competing as much as it was about developing the **competence** to complete the race in a reasonable amount of time.

Going back to my experience in the lab, I knew that the only thing I needed to do in order to achieve this goal was to determine what skills were needed and then come up with a plan to develop those skills. Whether it be weightlifting, powerlifting, Highland Games, obstacle course races, or flat-out endurance, the process is relatively simple:

1. Set a goal.
2. Determine the qualities necessary to complete the goal.
3. Assess what qualities you currently have and what you need to learn.
4. Design a plan that develops those qualities as efficiently as possible in the time given in a sequential manner.

(This last part is the most difficult part and does require some experience and insight, but overall, it is a simple process.)

So, what qualities did we need? We needed to be able to run three miles. We needed to be able to crawl through mud and under barbed wire. We needed to pull ourselves up and climb over walls, nets, and other structures. We started by running. We did some strength training. We practiced some of the skills we thought we would need for the obstacles such as climbing (pull-ups and monkey bars), crawling, and since we had to jump over fire at the end of the race, we practiced some jumping.

As an aside, we are social creatures and therefore social interaction can also be a very positive motivator.[126] Training with

126 João P. P. Rosa et al., ⬛Motivational and Evolutionary Aspects of a Phys-ical Exercise Training Program: A Longitudinal Study," *Frontiers in Psychology* 6: 648 (May 18, 2015).

friends and clients was an important part of this process. Exercising is far more tolerable if you have someone to talk to or suffer with, but there's a bit more to it than that.

It has been shown that we can actually begin to enjoy an activity simply by observing others enjoying the same activity. Additionally, those who have social support when exercising also tend to develop a better sense of self-efficacy and self-control.[127] Self-efficacy is a term that means having confidence in one's abilities to achieve one's goals. In other words, training with a supportive social group or partner gives us the confidence to say "Yes! I can do that!"

On race day, eight of us showed up to a farm in Pennsylvania that had been temporarily re-engineered into an obstacle course. Large structures dotted the rolling hills connected by broad muddy paths. Once we started, we were running and climbing for the better part of an hour. Everyone finished filthy, sore, exhausted, and elated. It was a great time, and all of us felt a little more accomplished at the end of the day, especially after finally getting all the mud out of our hair and ears.

---

127 Margie E. Lachman et al., "When Adults Don't Exercise: Behavioral Strategies to Increase Physical Activity in Sedentary Middle-Aged and Older Adults," *Innovation in Aging* 2, no. igy007 (April 5, 2018).

SETTING GOALS

Athletes and competitive types in general are highly motivated by competition, and it drives their performance.[128] That's great if you are an athlete or a competitive type. What if you feel you are not athletic? Or you lack the confidence to feel you can complete the task at hand? How do you reframe your thinking to allow yourself to succeed?

I found my motivation to get back to exercise by entering a competition. However, competition can be an incredible motivator for some and the complete opposite for others. This depends on whether people have a positive reaction to the competition, "I want to win," or a negative reaction, "I just don't want to be last."[129] Therefore, it is important, even when competing, **to set achievable and positive goals** for ourselves based on what we want to accomplish.

The kinds of goals you set make a difference in how well you stick to your program. Those who set goals based on mastery or the process of training (competence) tend to stick to their routines far longer than those who set goals based only on outcomes (appearance or rewards).[130] If you think about it, what we are trying to accomplish in exercise motivation is that you actually exercise, i.e., perform the behavior. If you are focused on an outcome of exercise such as losing weight, rather than reinforcing the actual behavior habit, you are less

---

128 João P. P. Rosa et al., "Motivational and Evolutionary Aspects of a Physical Exercise Training Program: A Longitudinal Study," *Frontiers in Psychology* 6: 648 (May 18, 2015).

129 Kou Murayama, "The Science of Motivation," American Psychology Association.

130 Ibid.

likely to continue the behavior.[131] Good habits take up to ten weeks to take hold, so it is important that we don't lose our motivation prematurely.[132]

Setting goals can include just about anything. Training is very much about the journey and not necessarily the destination. The goal itself is demonstration of the competence you have. For example, if your goal is to complete a 5K race, on race day, you are demonstrating that you can run five kilometers. Your training is what got you there.

My ultimate goal is to still be active enough to take my grandkids on long hikes, maybe take them for a surfing lesson, or get back on a horse or two well into my twilight years. The competitions may be fewer and farther between as I get older, but I'll always have something in mind that I'm working toward.

THE MOTIVATING POWER OF OTHER PEOPLE

One of the thought leaders in promoting fitness and trainer education in the US is Dr. Sal Arria. He had a vision as far back as the 1970s that would eventually launch the phenomenon of making personal training available to the masses. As a chiropractor for some of the top athletes in the world, Dr. Arria felt that strength training was the key to getting the

---

131 Wilson and Brookfield, "Effect of Goal Setting on Motivation and Adherence in a Six-Week Exercise Program,": 95–98.

132 Benjamin Gardner, Phillippa Lally, and Jane Wardle, "Making Health Habitual: The Psychology of 'Habit-Formation' and General Practice," *The British Journal of General Practice : The Journal of the Royal College of General Practitioners* 62, no. 605 (December 2012): 665–66.

injured athletes he worked with back on the field, stronger and more capable than before their injuries. He also felt that everyone deserved to benefit from that same knowledge, so he launched the International Sports Sciences Association (ISSA) with Fred Hatfield in 1988.[133]

In one of my many conversations with Dr. Arria, he told me that one of the reasons he founded the ISSA was because he knew that people needed help getting into and staying in an active lifestyle. He credited his own training partners over the years for getting him out of the office and into the gym when he was too focused on work. He thought that everyone should have someone to hold their hand and help them be accountable to what their bodies needed to be healthy. As social animals, socializing with others can be a powerful tool to break us out of our routine and do something that may be a bit uncomfortable for a while.

I would be lying if I told you it wasn't more fun to work out with other people. As I mentioned above, training for the Warrior Dash was far more fun since I had other people to suffer with. Group training can be a positive motivator, so I would encourage you to find a workout buddy or group you can meet up with for walks, runs, strength training sessions, bike rides, etc. Lately, I've noticed more people reporting that they are using Zoom, Facetime, or even just phone calls to work out together, though not physically, with their friends.

---

133 Sara Fleming, "From the 1984 Olympics to the Founding of the ISSA", *ISSA* (blog).

A 2015 article in the *British Journal of Sports Medicine* reviewing the benefits of outdoor walking groups demonstrated that the benefits of belonging to one of these groups went far beyond simply making people more physically active. There were improved measures with regard to blood pressure, resting heart rate, BMI, quality of life, and even depression. Additionally, these groups had a low drop-out rate, a high adherence rate, and virtually no negative effects.[134]

Safety is another concern that can be mitigated by training with others. Walking or running outdoors with others is safer than walking alone for any number of reasons. If you have concerns about balance or form when working out with weights, another set of eyes is always helpful. When you are not alone, there will always be someone there with a cell phone in case of an emergency.

SHOULD YOU HIRE A TRAINER OR COACH?

I think it's always a good idea to periodically hand the reins over to someone else, especially if you don't have a workout partner or group and need some accountability. This doesn't have to be prohibitively expensive. There are many trainers who work with small groups and others who will just check in with you online or on the phone once a week to help you stay on track with your diet and training. In fact, many fitness apps such as Peloton and Noom can help keep you motivated with live fitness class instructors and coaches who help you incorporate more healthy habits.

---

134 Sarah Hanson and Andy Jones, "Is There Evidence That Walking Groups Have Health Benefits? A Systematic Review and Meta-Analysis," *British Journal of Sports Medicine* 49, no. 11 (June 1, 2015): 710.

I have used coaches for a variety of reasons. The primary reason is when I don't know what I'm doing. Before I became a weightlifting coach, I hired a weightlifting coach to teach me correct technique. When I was struggling in the Highland Games, I hired a throwing coach to again, teach me correct technique. When I have needed to shed some pounds and had some trouble reining in my diet on my own, I have hired a nutrition coach.

Many clients come train with me for reasons beyond just managing their workouts. I've had them come for technique training on certain lifts, supervision on more difficult workouts, and simply to design a diet and exercise program they could do at home while checking in with me periodically.

If you are feeling a bit lost in terms of motivation and accountability, reach out to a few trainers in your area or online and see what they have to offer. In choosing a good trainer, you want one who listens to you, gives you good feedback, and helps you accomplish your goals.

WHAT ARE YOUR GOALS?

Going forward, it's time to think about setting some goals for yourself. What would you like to see yourself doing in three months, six months, a year from now, ten years from now? Are your goals related to lifestyle? Body composition? Recreational athletics? Competitions?

The most important variable in your training plan is time. Some goals may seem out of your reach, but with enough time and patience, most are reasonably attainable. If anyone had told me twenty years ago that I would be running a half-marathon, competing as a figure competitor, or competing in Highland Games in my forties, I would have thought they were crazy. Time and patience allowed me to build the fitness base and *competence* to make all those goals within my reach.

To get started with goal setting, think about how you would answer the following questions:

What things are easy for you to do?

Think about this in terms of the things that you do on a daily basis that don't involve strain or pain. These are things such as walking your dog, loading and unloading groceries from your car, loading and unloading kids and sports equipment, mowing the grass, doing basic yard work, playing with your kids, etc. It's okay if your list is short. For people with chronic back or joint pain, nothing may be easy. This is also a good time to think about your diet. Is it easy for you to have healthy foods at most meals?

What things are hard for you to do?

This list may be a little harder to make, it's not fun to focus on our shortcomings. Be honest though. I promise that the more things we identify, the more likely we are to improve them. If you have back or joint pain, what activities bother you the most? Do you get out of breath easily when walking or going up stairs? Do you fatigue easily when doing house or yard work? Have you backed out of activities with friends when you weren't confident you could participate? Again, let's take a look at diet. Is it difficult for you to have healthy foods at most meals?

What do you want to do better?

Think of three things you would like to do better. It can be something specific such as you'd like to start walking or running regularly. It can be something more general such as being able to get up out of a chair or your bed more easily. It might be focusing on your diet or joining a recreational league sport. Maybe you want to build a garden in your backyard. Maybe you want to take your grandkids hiking or keep up with them at Disney World. The important thing here is to write these goals down and put them somewhere that you will see them or be reminded of them regularly. I often put my goals in my training log, or I'll write them on a small piece of paper that I keep in my wallet.

* * *

My goal is to change the way you see your fitness journey. The worst thing we can do to ourselves is give up before we've started. Change takes time, and we must be patient. We must be open to new ways of thinking about exercise and fitness. We need to stop seeing exercise as punishment; instead, we need to regard it as what it really is, powerful and cheap medicine that is guaranteed to deliver better health and a better quality of life. As is the case with all medicines, it only works if we take it regularly.

CHAPTER 10

OVERCOMING YOUR FEAR AND ACHIEVING YOUR GOALS

———

When I step onto the field to compete in Highland Games, I'm rarely calm. I am nervous about performing well, I am nervous about hurting myself, I am nervous about losing. When it's time for the caber event, where we pick up a sixty-to-ninety-pound, fourteen-to-eighteen-foot standing log and try to turn it over, I am usually so anxious that I actually start to lose my balance. My feet don't feel connected to the earth, and I start to lose my peripheral vision.

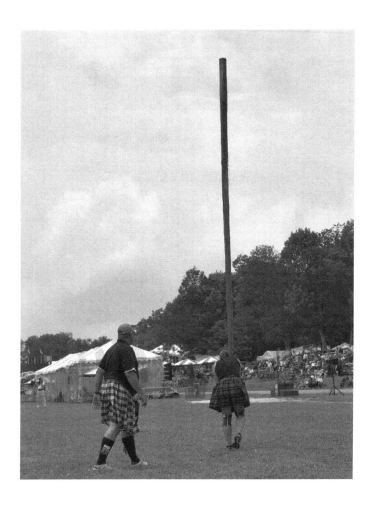

Figure 10.1: Caber

Fear used to keep me from doing a lot of the things I was drawn toward. As I related in the introduction, exerting myself rarely resulted in a graceful performance. Anxiety is something I have dealt with all my life and harnessing it has been a lifetime struggle. I realized a long time ago that I did not want fear ruling my life and have had to figure out ways to get around it. For me, and for the people I train, it comes down to meeting that fear head-on and running right through it with one of the most effective tools we have at our disposal: a plan.

When I step onto the field to compete in Highland Games, I've been training for weeks, if not months. I know I can lift and throw all the weights. I know I can pick up a caber. I can walk with one, I can run with one, and if it starts to fall while I'm holding it, I can get out from under it safely. I know this because I've been practicing. My brain may decide at the last minute that it does not want to be there, but my body knows what to do and is conditioned to handle the stress.

HOW TO MAKE A PLAN

By now, you should have a good understanding of how to design a program for everyday fitness. However, you may be wondering how we plan for a long-term specific goal? In the last chapter, I explained how I planned to train for the Warrior Dash by determining the specific requirements of the race. This concept of training for the specific requirements of an event or activity is the cornerstone of most athletic development programs. That may sound intimidating; however, it is no different from your initial assessment and program design except for now you have a timeline and possibly some new skills to learn.

The very first step is going to be to decide on a goal.

When setting a fitness goal, be specific. Do you want to improve your current fitness level, try a new skill or sport, focus on your body composition, or train for a specific event? I have helped people train for 5Ks, 10Ks, marathons, weight-lifting competitions, obstacle course races, CrossFit Regionals, and pre-season sports conditioning. However, there are many other goals to choose from that have nothing to do with formal competitions or events. I have also helped people train to get their first real pull-up, their first real push-up, be able to walk three miles without stopping, and regain their ability to walk up stairs without hanging onto the railing.

In order to evaluate your goal and how to approach it, we are going to take a similar approach to what we did in Chapter Three and perform an assessment. The next six questions will help you figure out what areas you need to focus on as well as how to determine a realistic timeline.

Do you need any rehab work or attention to a problem joint/muscle?

This may be an ongoing problem that just needs special attention as you train for your goal. Focusing on it during your warm-ups, spending some extra time stretching, or making sure to do some specific strength training are all ways we can keep our problem areas in mind.

We don't ever want to train through actual pain; however, we can work around our problem areas in a number of ways. No one is perfect one hundred percent of the time, and if we waited until we were 100 percent perfect to exercise, most of us would never get off the couch. Modify what you can, find stretches and movements that improve your mobility and coordination, and if necessary, see a physical therapist or other professional who can help you address the problem.

How strong do you need to be?

There is such a thing as "strong enough." Training to get as strong as possible has its place if you are a strongman, weightlifter, or powerlifter. Otherwise, there is a limit as to how strong you need to be in order to perform a task well. Training beyond that limit has a tendency to raise your risk of injury and negatively impact recovery. For example, if you are training to run a 5K, some full-body strength training with just your body weight or light implements will help you maintain your posture and protect your joints. However, regular *heavy* strength training while also trying to increase your running speed and/or distance can leave you too sore or fatigued to do either well.

How much endurance or aerobic fitness do you need?

Any activity that takes you longer than an hour to complete will benefit a great deal from some endurance and aerobic training. Obviously if you are training for an endurance event (walking, running, biking, swimming, etc.), the bulk of your training will take the form of whatever activity you are training for; specificity is important. However, with other activities, aerobic training has the hidden advantage of strengthening your stamina. Stamina is the ability to keep going over long periods of time, and it can provide a great advantage in both practice and competitive play.

I coached cross country and lacrosse when my kids were in middle school, and my youngest son participated in both sports. It took some patience and self-reflection for him to learn after two seasons of both sports that running cross country gave him the conditioning and stamina to be able to keep up with the other players in both lacrosse practices and games. In fact, despite not being the best technique-wise, he got more play time due to the fact he did not tire and could play consistently for the duration of the game. Since lacrosse is a running sport, developing running endurance is more helpful than non-specific aerobic training such as swimming or rowing; however, both of those exercises are far better than nothing.

It does not matter how good you are at a particular sport if you get fatigued before the period is over. Think about boxing and how much fighters rely on conditioning in addition to their fight skills. Tired boxers lose matches no matter how hard they can punch.

What are your strengths?

The biggest mistake people make when training for a goal is disregarding the fitness qualities that enabled them to start training to begin with. Some qualities erode more quickly than others. When training for endurance events, I have been known to stop weight training. Guess what happens when I stop squatting? My knees start hurting. I don't need to squat heavily or often—I *do* need to devote some time to squatting at least once a week if I want to run pain-free.

Likewise, when I was training CrossFit athletes, many of them came from endurance-based sports backgrounds such as soccer or swimming. They initially enjoyed a huge boost in performance from adding strength training and high-intensity interval training to their already enormous aerobic base. Unfortunately, over time that big aerobic base they built from doing high-volume aerobic work would begin to erode. Their progress would stall and sometimes regress. The simple solution was to replace a workout or two with some high-volume, low-intensity cardio, which always did the trick.

How will your everyday activities contribute to your goal?

This question is another one that many people tend to overlook. I once saw a blog article by a well-known fitness guru who was trying to make a point about not needing cardio if you regularly strength train. He pointed to his resting heart rate and blood pressure as proof of this argument. In that same blog article, he also mentioned that he lived in a large city and that he did not drive.

When I pressed him on how much he actually walked, he admitted he probably walked a total of four to five miles a day just going to work, to the market, and to social events. There is a big difference between someone who sits at a desk all day and drives to and from work versus someone who is on and off their feet all day, such as a nurse or a delivery person. How do your daily activities enhance your strength, endurance, aerobic fitness, and stamina?

How much time do you have to train?

The most important part of your goal is WHEN the goal is to be completed and HOW OFTEN you have to train. It's important that you set a realistic timeline that allows you to safely acquire the strength, endurance, aerobic fitness, and skills necessary to complete the goal. For example, if I were to train for a half-marathon again, I would have to consider myself a beginner and give myself a full six months to reach that goal.

I would say, in general, that most people can make significant progress toward a goal in about twelve to sixteen weeks if they are training three to four days per week. The newer you are to the activity, the more time you need. That's about thirty-six to sixty-four training sessions in total. Since you are keeping a training log, you should have a good idea as to how quickly you can make progress and how much recovery you need. Use this hindsight to help you determine a reasonable timeline.*

* *As an experienced coach, I still need to observe someone for at least a month or two as well as have an accurate understanding of their training history before I can target specific timeline goals, so remember to cut yourself some slack and be patient.*

THE PLANNING PROCESS

Now that you've evaluated your goal, it's time to come up with a plan. This plan does not have to be overly complicated, and at the most basic level simply provides you with the skills you need to complete your goal. As I stated in the beginning, when I am preparing to compete in the Highland Games, I need to make sure I have enough postural and joint strength to prevent injury and enough practice with the implements to perform well. I can't account for everything, however. For example, one time I was walking with a caber, slipped on some mud, and landed on my back. Thankfully, the caber went the other way.

The following visual is my attempt to simplify goal planning to three separate phases. I will make it even simpler by telling you that most fitness goals only require the first step, "base and rehab."

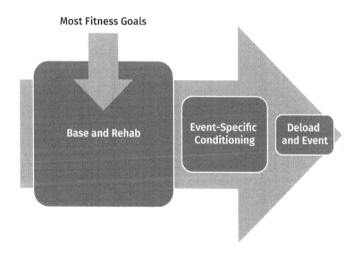

"**Base and rehab**" is the biggest part of everyone's training plan, whether they have a goal or not. For most people, your **base** is your foundational fitness, the strength and aerobic fitness which you continually work on and improve. **Rehab**

refers to more specific exercises that focus on problem areas to either improve old injuries or prevent new ones.

When you have a specific goal in mind, your base will include the specific demands of that goal. For example, if you want to be a basketball player, your base will include your strength and aerobic foundational fitness activities as well as basketball practice. If you want to run a 5K, your base will include running and some supportive strength training. If you want to compete in a powerlifting meet, your primary activities will consist of learning and practicing technique on the squat, bench press, and deadlift and some supportive aerobic training.

What you should see in the above paragraph is that all three scenarios have aerobic training, strength training, and specific skill training. However, these activities take on different priorities based on the goal.

How much base is enough?

You just want enough of a base that you can have fun and not get hurt. I like to think of base development and rehab as something that is always going on in the background that supports the activities we want to participate in. For most people, this phase is ongoing and can be the foundation of training for most events. If you want to throw some pick-up basketball, rec league soccer, or some weekend hikes on top of your regular training, go for it. Like I said, as long as you can keep up, have fun, and not get hurt, there is no reason not to. Below you will see how I modified my base/rehab phase to help me prepare for a vacation that was all about hiking.

The **"event-specific conditioning"** phase strictly applies to more specialized events that require a specific skill set and/or an emphasis on either strength or endurance. It also depends on the level of performance you want to achieve. A person who wants to complete a 5K and doesn't care about their time probably does not need this phase, whereas someone who wants to set a personal record is going to want to focus more specifically on just running during the last several weeks before the race. When I am training powerlifters, I have them focus primarily on lifting and recovery during the eight weeks leading up to their competition. Pre-season sports practices are another example of this strategy. If your fitness base is established, it's time to turn it into something useful on the field.

The difference between this phase and the base/rehab phase is that a general fitness approach will not deliver the specific strength and/or conditioning you need to perform well in your specific event or activity. If you want to be good at basketball, you have to practice playing basketball.

The important thing to remember about this phase is that you need to ensure you aren't piling it on top of what you are already doing. It's okay to replace some regular workouts or aerobic exercise with some sports practice or specific training. Once you get into the swing of things, you will have a better idea of if and when you can add some things back in. I learned the hard way that training for a half-marathon on top of my throwing/lifting schedule was a terrible idea even though I felt pretty good the first few months. Don't be like me.

Generally speaking, if you have a good fitness base in place, event-specific conditioning time periods can be as short as four weeks and as long as twelve weeks. Team sports typically only practice for four to six weeks before the season begins. Most strength sports have an eight-week peaking period. Endurance sports have a little bit longer peaking period, usually twelve weeks. For most beginner-level activities, four to eight weeks is plenty.

The **"deload and event"** phase is short and really only applies to single events. A few days or even a week off to recover fully and mentally prepare before competition is always a good thing. Some light activity and stretching during that time is a great idea, but we are talking intensities and durations of less than fifty percent of what you've been doing. It is common for people to be afraid that if they take time off, they will lose all their progress. I can assure you this does not happen. I have never seen anyone fail to perform well after a deload. I have, however, seen people bomb out completely when they pushed themselves too hard that last few days before competition.

HIKING IN THE SOUTHWEST

In 2018, my husband and I planned to take our kids to the Southwestern United States for Spring Break. We planned to visit several national parks in Utah and Arizona including Bryce Canyon, Zion, Arches, Sedona, and the Grand Canyon, which would require two to six hours of hiking each day. I had just gotten back to regular training after taking several months off after my half-marathon. If you recall, I had developed rather painful plantar fasciitis, and unfortunately, this condition also resulted in knee pain, which made walking up and down stairs rather painful. So, as you can imagine, I was a bit anxious about hiking in places with big hills.

In answering the questions above, I had the following answers:

1. **Do you need any rehab or attention to a problem joint/ muscle?** My knees were going to need a great deal of rehabilitation. I spoke with my chiropractor, and he thought that I needed to work on stretching my glutes (specifically my glute medius) as well as my quads. It took me a little while to figure out the right combination, and I eventually found that adding in some light quad extensions and banded sidewalks (see Appendix B) to my warm-up exercises before squatting or deadlifting helped reduce soreness and knee pain in general after my workouts. A combination of stretching and strengthening my quads and gluteus medius in addition to strengthening my hips and legs in general seemed to do the trick. After three to four months, stairs were no longer scary to me.

2. **How strong do you need to be?** Hiking is a bit different than walking, especially if you are carrying a pack. You need full-body strength, especially in your legs, core, and upper back, so a regular strength routine was important to include. My program included squats, push-ups, deadlifts, rows, core work, and a variety of shoulder exercises. As you may recall from Chapter One, strength is the foundation of endurance, and hip and leg strength were especially important for the hiking I would be doing.

3. **How much endurance or aerobic fitness do you need?** I didn't have any mountains to hike in Raleigh. I did have a treadmill with an incline setting. I needed both specific endurance (hiking) as well as a boost to my general

aerobic endurance to give me some stamina, so I would try and walk on an incline thirty to forty-five minutes, three to four days per week. Stamina is an incredibly important part of completing an event or activity, and hiking requires a great deal of stamina. Four miles on a track may only take you an hour to complete. A hiking trail is a different story. For example, a popular hike at the Grand Canyon is the South Kaibab Trail to Cedar Ridge. The round-trip distance for this hike is only two point eight miles, but it takes most people two to three hours to complete. I'll tell you from personal experience that the hike back up is way more challenging than the way down. It's not the time you want to be losing steam.

4. **What are your strengths?** My biggest strength is my posture. I've never really lost that postural strength developed through hours of riding horses when I was younger, and it's been reinforced over the years by always moving with good posture. However, carrying a pack was going to require more upper-back and shoulder strength to stay upright. In addition to rows, I also added in some reverse flies and face pulls to my program (see Appendix B).

5. **How will your everyday activities contribute to your goal?** My daily activities actually keep me on my feet quite a bit, especially when coaching sports. I would be coaching lacrosse two months prior to leaving for Spring Break, and that meant I would be on my feet, moving around for about two hours a day, five days a week. This extra exercise would contribute to my overall stamina as well.

6. **How much time do you have to train?** My schedule was pretty packed, especially in the afternoons when I was coaching sports, making dinner, helping with homework,

and catching up with my students and clients. I started going to bed earlier and waking up an hour early to get my workouts in. Since I had started training for this trip six months out, my inability to train for longer periods every other day didn't really impact my results. This wasn't a competition, rather, it was just about being able to hike up and down some canyons without hurting myself while also having fun with my family. Patience is the most important part of goal setting and a lot of people derail their progress by being too ambitious with their timelines. *A good rule to keep in mind is to take your first estimation of how much time you may need between starting and achieving a goal and double it.*

Overall, this goal was relatively simple to achieve and just involved re-establishing my fitness base and rehabbing my knees. I did take into account that I would need to be on my feet and moving for several hours a day. For what it's worth, I took a similar approach several years prior when my husband and I took our three children to Disney World, and I knew I would be carrying a backpack, pushing a stroller, maybe carrying a child, and possibly doing all three while running to catch a shuttle.

My **base and rehab** for this goal were simply full body strength, incline walking endurance, and paying special attention to my knees. Had I been more motivated, I could have probably taken some weekend trips to the mountains for some **event-specific conditioning**. I didn't have time in my schedule for these mountain outings, so incline treadmill walks had to serve this purpose.

One more thing to consider in all this planning is what event-specific equipment and clothing you are going to need. For this trip, it was just going to be good shoes and socks, clothing that did not rub, and an ergonomic water pack. Hydration is incredibly important, especially in arid country at high elevations.

Since this was a general fitness goal, I did not necessarily need a **deload**. I do always think it is a good idea not to hurt yourself before sitting on a plane or in a car for several hours, so the last few days before our trip, I just focused on stretching and some long walks.

* * *

One of the things that was surprising to me as I started accomplishing my goals was how I felt when I completed them. I thought I would feel an elevated sense of achievement or pride. I thought I would realize some newfound confidence or feel particularly elated. What I found instead was that the feelings of achievement, pride, confidence, and elation actually occurred on the way to the goal. When you train correctly, what you achieve on the day of your competition or event is already known to you. What you should feel when you step onto the field, the starting line, or wherever your challenge lies is "I've got this." Because you do. It is precisely what you've been practicing for.

EPILOGUE

The amount of information in this book may seem over-whelming. Don't worry, you don't have to use it all at once. It's okay if you want to spend a few months just increasing your daily activity by walking and being more active throughout your day. If you add strength training to your routine, it is perfectly fine if you don't move past the exercises in Chapter Six for a while. I want you to take the lessons in this book at your own pace and incorporate them as you are able. One thing I know to be true about habits is that if we try to incorporate too many of them into our routines at once, we have a hard time keeping any of them.

"He who hunts two hares catches neither."

ADAGIA, *ERASMUS*

That being said, I will leave you with some final thoughts to apply to your fitness journey. You can travel this road for as long as you like, at a speed of your own choosing, and I wish you great success.

Everything Is a Skill

When you treat training as skill development, end points become much easier to recognize, i.e., when form breaks down, the session is over. Whether you are strength training, walking or running, or just throwing a ball back and forth, when form, energy, accuracy, etc. begin to diminish, end the session or switch to something else.

Have a Plan

Having a plan keeps things simple. Build your plan around simple goals. Have a plan for each day as well as a weekly template or set of goals. This plan can be as simple as a short list of fitness goals you want to hit that week, such as walking a total of five miles, completing two circuit training sessions, taking a yoga class, etc. When you consider the demands of work, school, family, friends, and house chores, plans should be as simple as possible. Don't forget, yard work and walking or biking for transportation are exercise!

Be Ready to Adjust Your Plan

Our schedules are unpredictable. There is a meme that says something to the effect of "adulthood is constantly saying 'after this week, everything will get easier' until you die." That's not untrue. Cut yourself some slack, and if you are having a hard time regularly sticking with your plan, it's probably a good idea to come up with a new plan.

"Train" All Year

Whether this means playing different sports throughout the year or taking the summer off to spend more time walking your dog or your kids, the goal is to stay active in some capacity throughout the year. Think broadly about training. What

I mean by training is broad balanced activity that expresses your physicality. Year-round physical activity is good for you. This does not mean you need formal structured training all year but staying active will keep you relatively strong and conditioned for whatever activities you enjoy. Keep it fun.

Prioritize Recovery

We often lack the ability to know when we've done too much until we've done too much, too often. Although motivation for some of us can be a problem, for others, the opposite can be a problem. Take an honest look at how much you are doing both physically and mentally. All of it adds up.

Pay Attention to Pain and Fatigue

Overuse injuries often don't rear their ugly head until they become acute and affect your daily life. Make a note of any aches and pains in your training log and what activities tend to make them worse.

Proper Fuel

I did not address diet in the main chapters of this book because I think exercise deserves its own spotlight. However, our diets are intrinsically linked to our body composition and health. Appendix B contains some basic dietary infor-mation as well as some less well-known information on why we have a tendency to overeat. It also has some strategies for approaching your diet in a way that is healthy, sustainable, and most importantly, delicious.

Enjoy Yourself!

The main reason for improving our fitness, as I see it, is so we can get out and enjoy life more with our families and friends for as long as we are here. Whether you enjoy playing pick-up basketball, dancing, or just taking long walks in the woods, remember that your quality-of-life matters. Fitness can give us independence and access to some pretty amazing places and activities. One of the best ways to stay motivated to stay fit for life is to find the things that bring you joy and do them regularly.

Whose woods these are I think I know.
His house is in the village though;
He will not see me stopping here
To watch his woods fill up with snow.

My little horse must think it queer
To stop without a farmhouse near
Between the woods and frozen lake
The darkest evening of the year.

He gives his harness bells a shake
To ask if there is some mistake.
The only other sound's the sweep
Of easy wind and downy flake.

The woods are lovely, dark and deep,
But I have promises to keep,
And miles to go before I sleep,
And miles to go before I sleep.

Stopping by Woods on a Snowy Evening
Robert Frost

APPENDIX A

ADDITIONAL EXERCISES
AND STRETCHES

———

The activities below are additional exercises for each body section named in Chapter Five. The explanations will be briefer as the main exercises have already been exhaustively broken down. Keep in mind the form points explained in Chapters Five and Six. If you have access to YouTube, you can find video instruction for virtually all these exercises on multiple channels as well as a few variations for each. Remember, it is the movement itself that matters.

These are by no means an exhaustive list of all available exercises for your body. You can find all kinds of exercises on the internet that claim to be the best for x, y, and z, but I think it's a good idea to be conservative when building a foundational program.

CORE EXERCISES

Crunches and **sit-ups** are two of the most common abdominal exercises that people think of when training their core. To properly perform a crunch, you want to be thinking about keeping your neck neutral and lifting your shoulders and upper back off the floor.

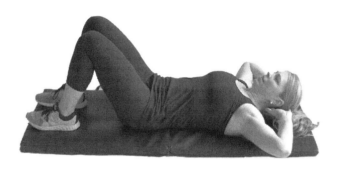

Crunch 1

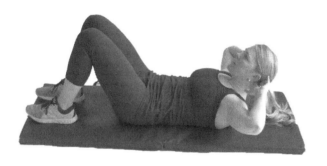

Crunch 2

Ordinary sit-ups are an exercise I don't prescribe very often. If you anchor your feet, you are primarily using your hip flexors instead of your core muscles, and if you don't anchor your feet, you can sometimes do some damage to your low back as it may excessively flex and extend during the movement. One solution is to place a rolled-up towel under your low back to provide some support. The other solution is to perform your sit-up with a weight of some kind, I prefer a medicine ball. The **medicine ball sit-up** is similar to a goblet squat in that pushing the ball in front of you as you sit up helps displace the center of gravity of your upper body somewhat.

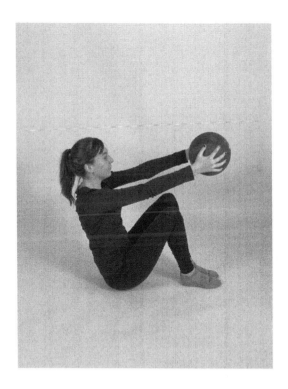

Medicine Ball Sit-up 1

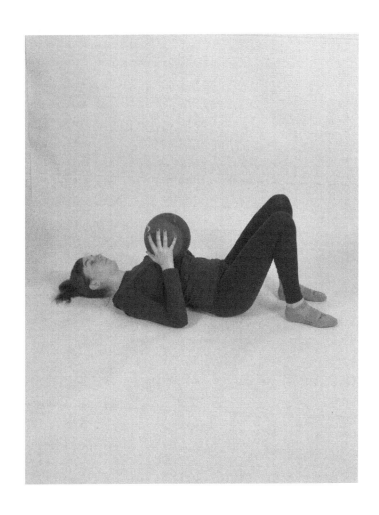

Medicine Ball Sit-up 2

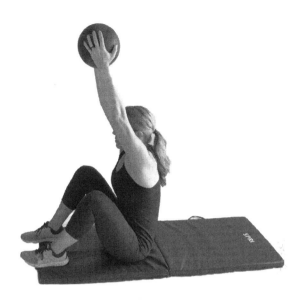

Medicine Ball Sit-up Overhead

A **plank** is essentially the start position of a push-up, and it can be performed either supporting your weight with your hands or down on your forearms. If you are very new to planks, you can do these from a raised surface or from your knees, too, as long as your body is in a straight line. I will add planks to a strength circuit by prescribing a certain amount of time for my trainees to hold it. For example, thirty, forty-five, or sixty seconds. Planks work well at the end of a circuit before the rest period.

Side planks target the core in a different way, as well as the shoulder. You can perform them with your arm up and chest open, or your arm down. The former is more difficult balance-wise. When using side planks, I will have my trainees alternate sides (and even add a regular plank in between) for short-timed intervals as above. This can be a stand-alone core "finisher" if you like, where you hold each position for thirty to sixty seconds and perform multiple rounds.

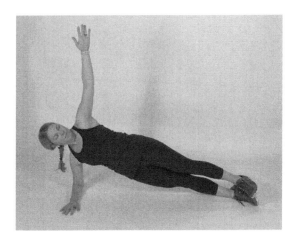

Side Plank 1

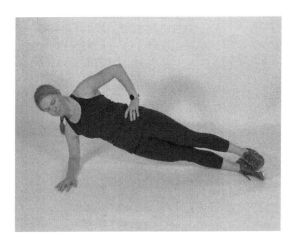

Side Plank 2

A **bird dog** is an exercise that is far more challenging than it looks. It is fatiguing to the shoulder, upper back, core, hips, and leg. You get down into an "all fours" position, on your hands and knees, and then lift your opposing arm and leg. Again, you will hold this position for thirty to sixty seconds before switching to the other side.

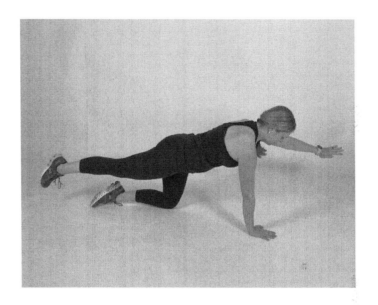

Bird Dog

A **superman** is a back and hip exercise that, like the plank and bird dog, is a position you hold for a set length of time. It is important that when performing this exercise, you try and get both your shoulders and chest as well as your thighs off the ground.

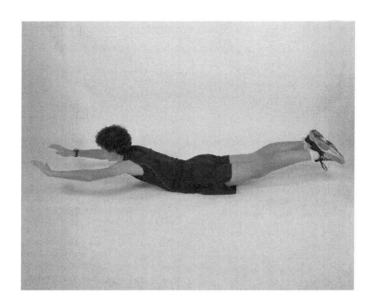

Superman

A **leg raise** is an exercise you can perform from the floor that targets your lower abdominal muscles. Notice that Elizabeth has her hands under her hips. This helps to stabilize her low back as she raises her legs.

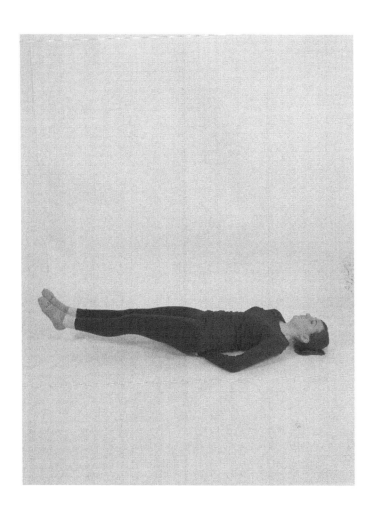

Leg Raise 1

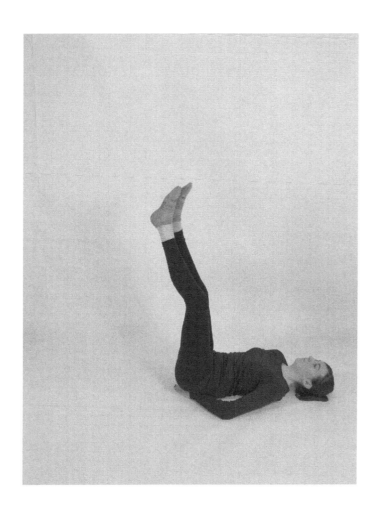

Leg Raise 2

If you have a pull-up bar or even some monkey bars to hang from, hanging knee raises are another great way to train your lower core. You simply pull your knees up as far as you can. You may notice your body starts to swing when you do these, so keep a chair that you can touch with your foot nearby to stop swinging. You can add some rotation to this by lifting your knees up while also rotating your hips to one side and alternating.

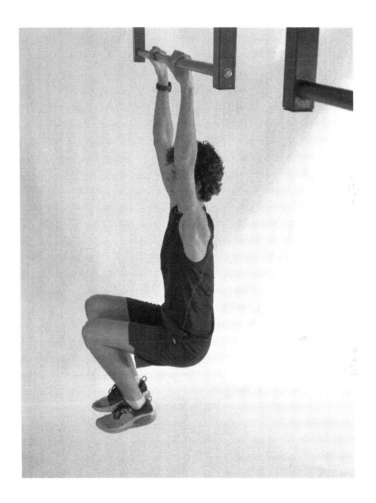

Hanging Knee Raises

A **wood chop** is essentially the same movement as the standing Russian twist except that you start with your weight down near your hip on one side and raise it to shoulder level as you rotate to the other side. It is a bit awkward to do these in a back-and-forth fashion, so I recommend you do one direction at a time, simply resetting between repetitions.

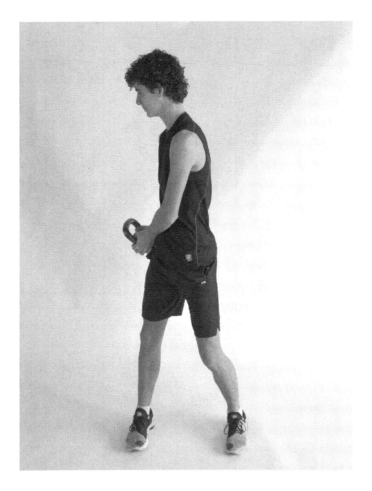

Wood Chop 1

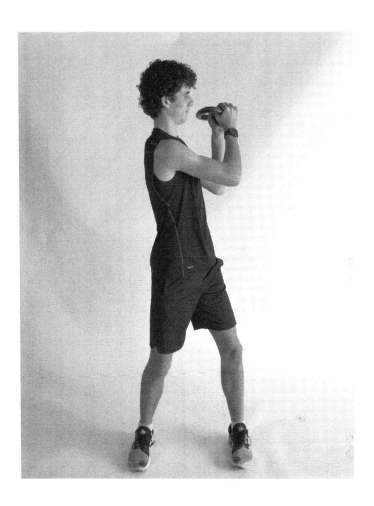

Wood Chop 2

CORE STRETCHES

The psoas is a deep hip flexor that attaches your femur to your spine just under your ribcage. When it is overly tight, it can actually cause your low back to hyperextend and cause low back pain. You can stretch this muscle in several ways, and the first is the **hurdler stretch**. In the photo, Elizabeth is stretching her psoas on the left side by leaning back in a lunge position. If this muscle is tight, you will feel it deep in your abdomen as you lean back.

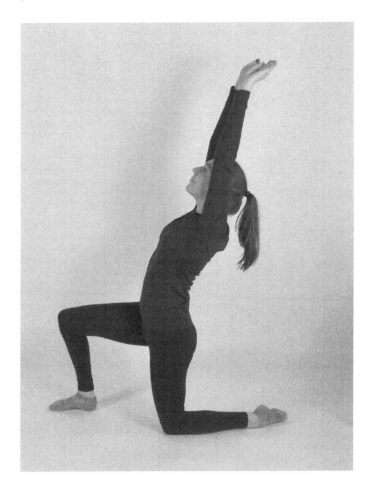

Hurdler Stretch

The **lying psoas stretch** is a good way to hit the top of the muscle. You simply lie flat on your back and place one arm straight up. You will simultaneously reach in opposite directions with both your hand and your foot. You will typically feel this stretch closer to your rib cage than your pelvis.

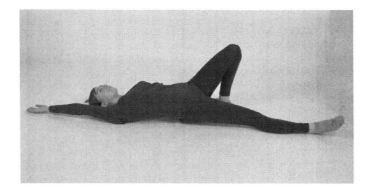

Lying Psoas Stretch

The **cat-cow stretch** are two separate positions that stretch both the back and neck muscles and the abdominal muscles. To start, get into an all-fours position. To get into **cat**, push your head down and arch your back upward like a Halloween cat. You should feel a nice stretch down the length of your spine from your head to your hips. To get into **cow**, reverse the position by lifting your head up and sinking your spine down below your hips and shoulder blades. You should feel a stretch across your belly and chest. Since these stretches are complementary, you can alternate between them with ten-to-thirty-second holds.

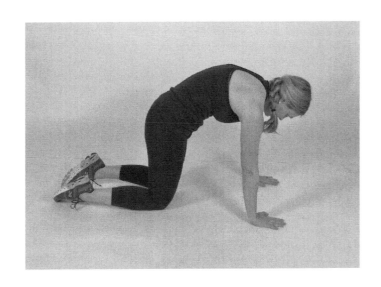

Cat

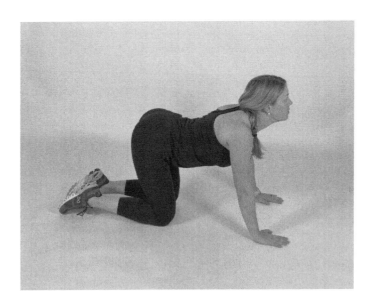

Cow

HIP AND LEG EXERCISES

I periodically have clients who have trouble squatting from time to time, so I have to introduce another exercise to flex and extend their knees. **Step-ups** are a good substitute. For this exercise you will need a raised surface such as an aerobic step, a box, or simply a stair step. You can do these exercises with weights or without. Simply place one foot on the box, shift your weight forward into the raised leg, and extend it until you are standing on the box. Step back down and repeat. For building strength, I recommend completing your reps on one leg before switching to the other. I would not use a box any higher than twelve inches for this exercise. If you have knee pain, make sure your knee isn't going too far forward as you step up, and keep your weight in your midfoot. You can also try using a lower box.

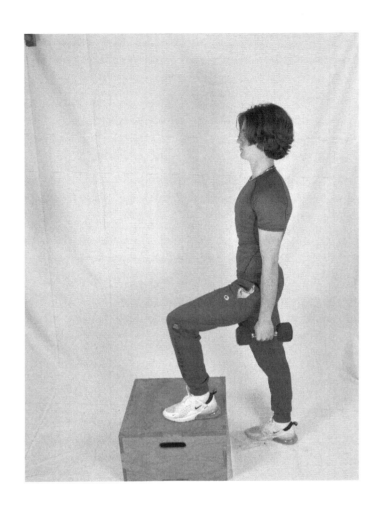

Step-ups 1

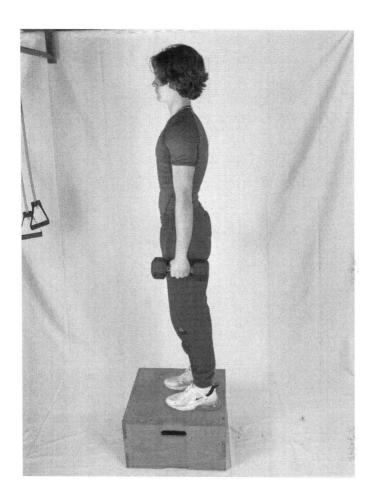

Step-ups 2

Lunges are another exercise that can be subbed in for squats. Do be careful with lunges as this is an exercise that can be helpful or harmful depending on how you do them.

The most important thing for you to keep in mind is that your knee does not extend beyond your toe. In the first photo,

Laura has stepped back from a standing position and lowered her back knee until it is almost at the floor. This is important, as you don't want your knee coming into contact with the floor. The depth you choose is up to you, as you may find it difficult to get that deep at first. What you may not notice in this picture is that her feet are still hip-width apart, i.e., they are not directly in line with one another. This is important for maintaining your balance.

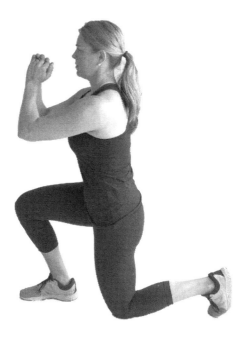

Lunge

You can step forward as you lunge and even do walking lunges where you walk forward and lunge on every step.

However, in walking forward, you may have more of a tendency to push your knee forward so be careful when using forward lunges.

Lunges can be multidirectional. In the next two photos, Laura is lunging to the side and also forward at a 45-degree angle. These different directions will affect your hips and knees differently, so they might make you sore in some different places.

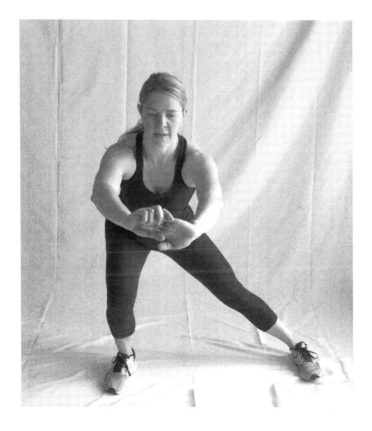

Side Lunge

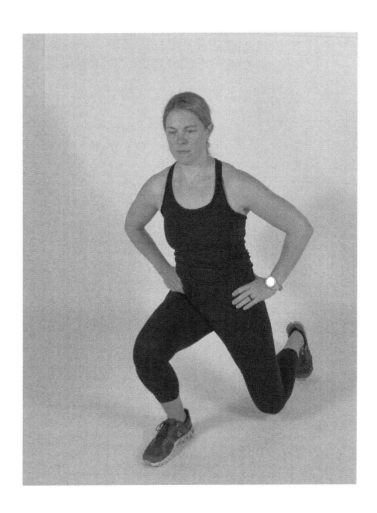

Diagonal Lunge

The split squat is very similar to the lunge, although there is only one step involved. You step back once and then execute your repetitions by raising and lowering your knee to the floor. This is a good solution for people who have trouble with balance. It is also a movement you can load significantly if using a barbell in a squat rack.

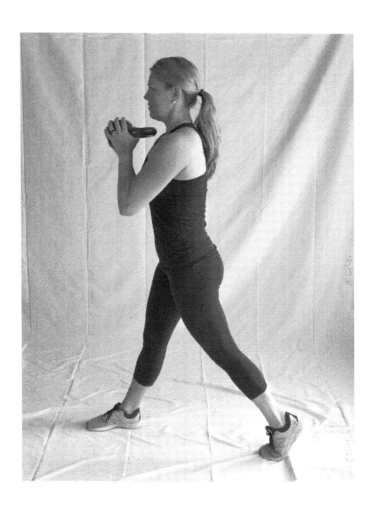

Split Squat 1

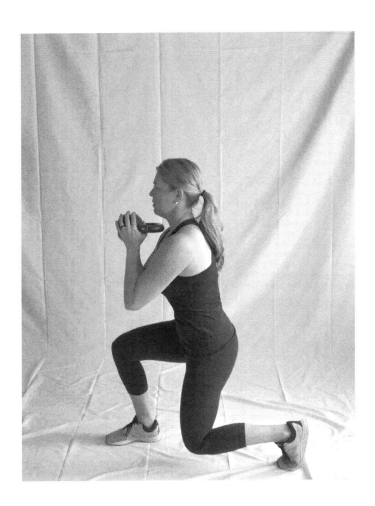

Split Squat 2

Hamstring curls are typically done in the gym with a machine. They can be difficult to replicate in a home gym, although one way to do them is with bands. The following photos demonstrate how you can do them with a stability ball. Hamstring curls are not terribly necessary except for some rehab work or bodybuilding.

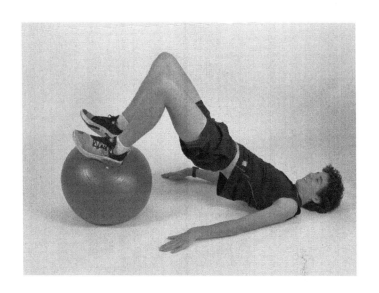

Hamstring Curls 1

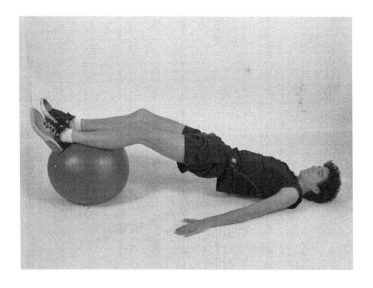

Hamstring Curls 2

Bridges are a simple way to target your hips, hamstrings, and lower back. You can perform this as a static hold, or you can begin with your hips resting on the ground and perform them with repetitions. Placing a dumbbell or a plate on your hips will add some resistance.

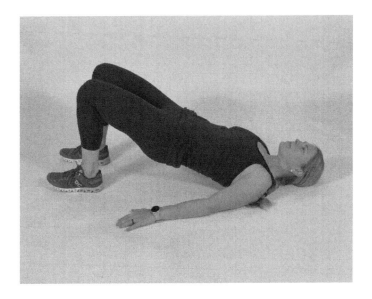

Bridges

Quad extensions, like hamstring curls, are another exercise that are typically done on a gym machine. Some people do not recommend them as they can cause stress on the knee. Personally, I do not care for them unless they are done with light weights, though they can serve a purpose in rehab or bodybuilding. One version of a quad extension is performed standing with a band anchored at a low position; it is called a "terminal knee extension" or TKE. You can easily find instructional videos on how to perform these extensions, but they are mostly considered a rehab exercise.

If you have a problem doing squats and have switched to step ups or lunges, you still need to strengthen that glute medius to help stabilize your knee. **Side walks with a band** are a great solution for this issue. For this, you will need a small band with light resistance or even a physical therapy band. You will place it around your lower leg anywhere from your ankle to knee. Place your feet under your hips and push your hips back as though you are about to deadlift, and then step sideways with one foot. I typically have people do ten steps in each direction for three to five sets. This is also a great warm-up to get your knee stabilizers working before going for a walk or run.

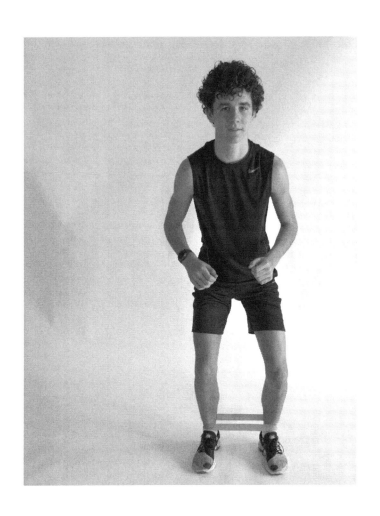

Side Walk with Band 1

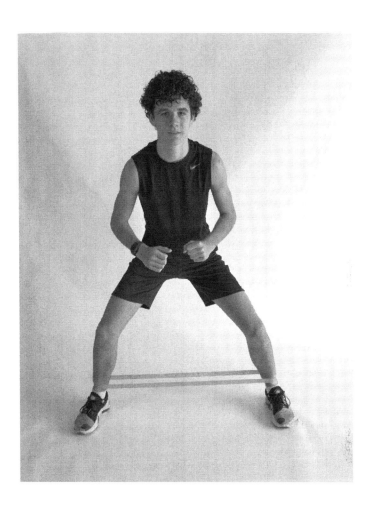

Side Walk with Band 2

Calf raises are something we should all do from time to time, and they are pretty simple to perform. You can do them on the floor or even on a step to get a bigger range of motion. To add more resistance, lift one leg so you are lifting all your bodyweight with one side or even hold on to a dumbbell. You can hold on to a wall or a broomstick for balance as needed.

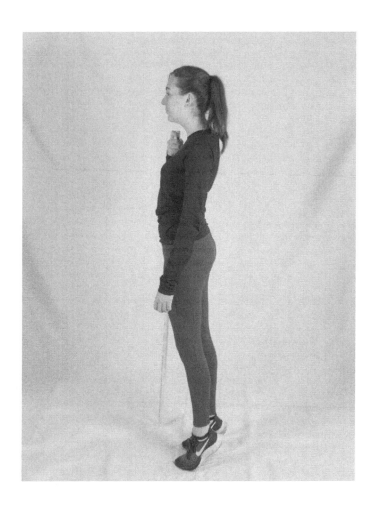

Calf Raises

HIP AND LEG STRETCHES

The cool-down stretches in Chapter Eight are largely for the lower back, hips, and legs, so start there.

The **Figure 4 stretch** is another stretch that targets the piriformis and helps open up the pelvis.

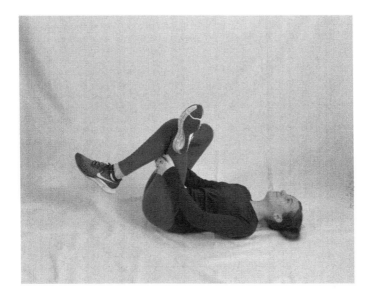

Figure 4 stretch

Child's pose is a yoga pose that helps stretch out the ankles, legs, and hips while relaxing the rest of the body. Sit down with your legs folded under you and your knees out in front. Push your knees apart and fold forward until your arms are stretched out in front of you, and your forehead is near or touching the floor.

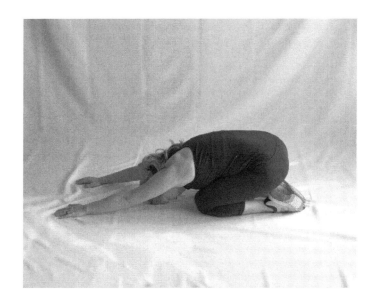

Child's Pose

Whether you train your calves or not, you will want to stretch them regularly. Tight calves can be a source of heel, foot, and knee pain. Kids going through growth spurts will often develop tight calves, which can cause Achilles tendonitis if not addressed. The simplest way to stretch your calves is to stand with the balls of your feet on the edge of a stair step and let your weight sink down into your heels.

In the **calf stretch** pictured, Elizabeth has her back toe on the floor and is stretching her calf by trying to press her heel to the floor.

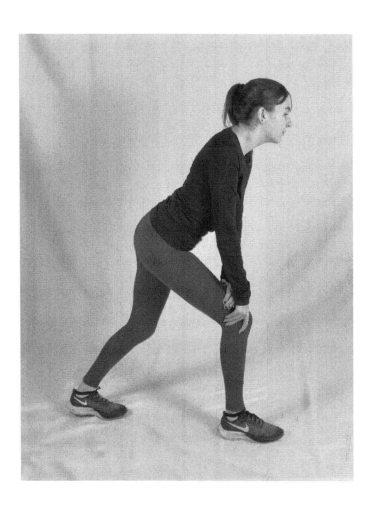

Calf Stretch

SHOULDER AND ARM EXERCISES

Shoulders can be delicate. As I stated in Chapter Five, they are largely held together by the surrounding muscles, tendons, and ligaments. Therefore, I think this shoulder complex is a nice addition to any program. It is done by performing all three exercises with very light weights, from soup cans to five-pound dumbbells, for sets of ten to fifteen reps. Three rounds are usually enough. I will have clients do this as part of their warm-up or cool-down. It does not have to be part of your strength circuit, although you could incorporate the individual exercises if you like.

The **front raise** begins with holding two dumbbells in front of you and simply raising your arms forward until they are parallel to the ground. **Side raises** are done the same way, but you raise your arms laterally. In the photo, Patrick has bent his arms 90 degrees at the start. Side raises can be stressful on the shoulder joint, especially if you have long arms, so decreasing the length of the lever by bending your arm reduces some of that stress. The last exercise, the **reverse fly**, targets the back of the shoulder. You start by pushing your hips back and bending forward as if to perform a row and then pulling your arms back until they are parallel with your torso. You can keep your arms straight for this exercise, but many people find it more comfortable if they bend their arms.

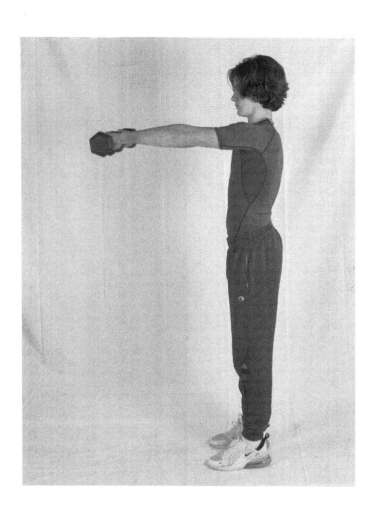

Front Raise

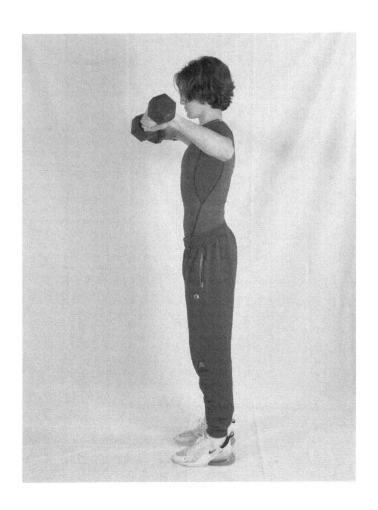

Side Raise

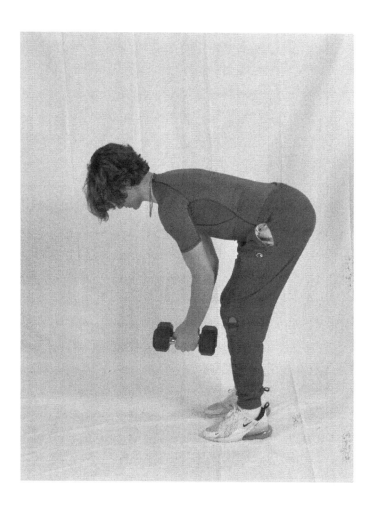

Reverse Fly

This is a very simple exercise for your triceps. Lean forward with your hips back as though you are going to row. Pull your upper arms in line with your torso and bend your elbows. You want to be leaning far enough forward that when you extend your arm, the weights are moving against gravity.

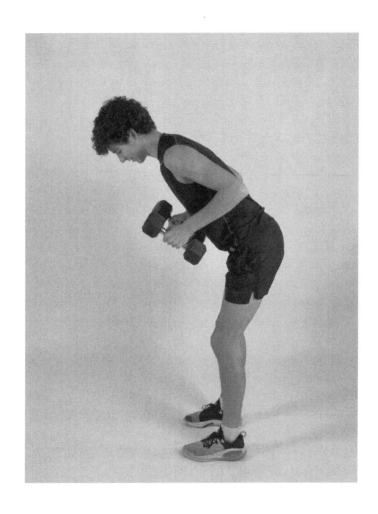

Triceps Kickback 1

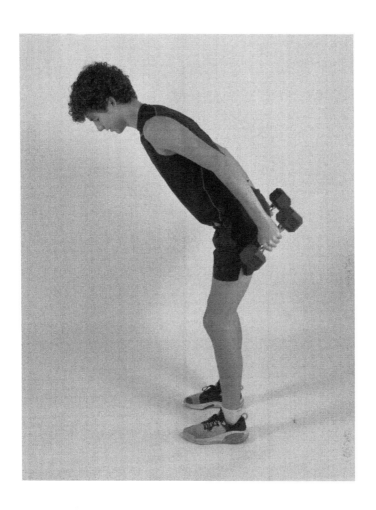

Triceps Kickback 2

Dips are an exercise that targets the triceps, but also the upper back and chest. The beginner version of **dips** is to do them with your feet on the floor and your hands behind you on a raised surface. You want your back to be nice and straight. As you lower yourself down by bending your arms, you want to keep your body as close to the raised surface as possible. If you get too far out in front, it can bother your shoulders.

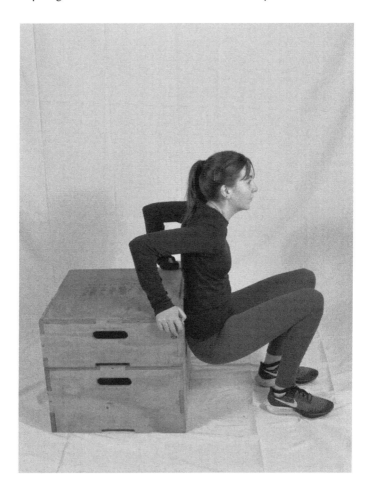

Bench Dip 1

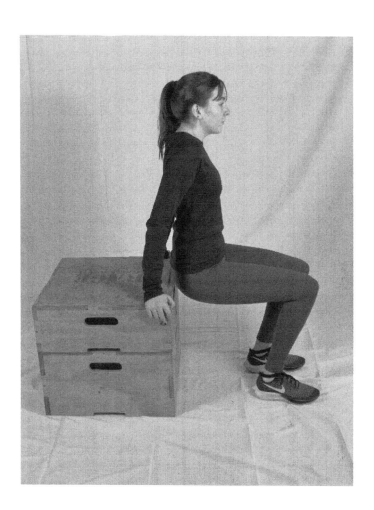

Bench Dip 2

I did not include pictures of **biceps curls** in this section. That does not mean you shouldn't be doing them. If you have triceps exercises included in your program, biceps exercises should be included as well.

CHEST AND BACK EXERCISES

When performed correctly, I love the **bench press**. However, I don't see it often being performed correctly in gyms or in YouTube videos. The bench press is a full-body exercise that allows you to lift weight off your chest through an arc of tension created from your upper back all the way down to your feet. This movement is what allows powerlifters to lift two or three times their bodyweight in the bench press. They aren't just using their chest and arms; they are using their whole body.

In the first picture, Elizabeth is not lying passively on the bench. Her feet are firmly in contact with the floor, her glutes are contracted, and her upper back and head are in contact with the bench. You may notice an arch in her low back as well. Since the low back is not loaded in this lift, this hyper-extension is okay. Her shoulder blades are pulled back and slightly down her back to create tension in her back that goes all the way down to her feet. Her elbows are out at about a 45-degree angle relative to her torso.

When she presses those dumbbells up, she is going to be pressing the dumbbells with her arms, pressing her feet against the floor, and pressing her butt and upper back against the bench. With that tension in her upper back, her shoulders are far more stable, and she can move more weight. The benefit of using dumbbells for the bench is that she can rotate her wrists to have a more neutral or pronated grip depending on her comfort.

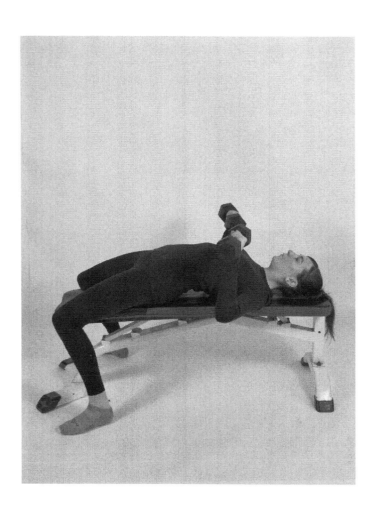

Bench Press 1

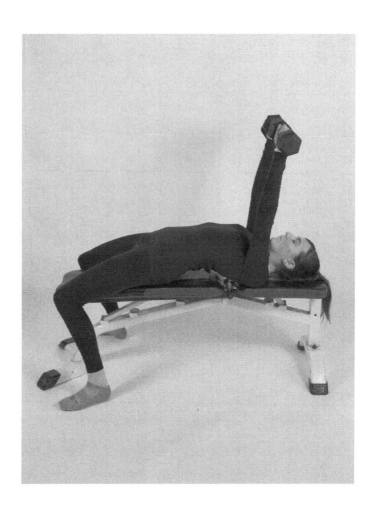

Bench Press 2

The **face pull** requires a band or a pulley system. This highly underrated exercise targets the very top of the upper back and has come to my rescue many times when my shoulders are a little too beat up from throwing. This is another exercise like the shoulder complex that can be done with little resistance and lots of reps. You can include it in a strength circuit or do it as a warm-up or cool-down exercise. In the photos, Elizabeth is doing a face pull with a resistance band attached to a pull-up bar. She starts with her arms out in front of her, up above her eyes. She then pulls the band straight back, keeping her arms and elbows raised, until her fists are in line with her ears.

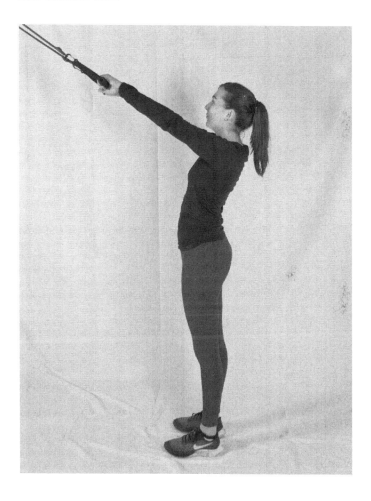

Face Pulls 1

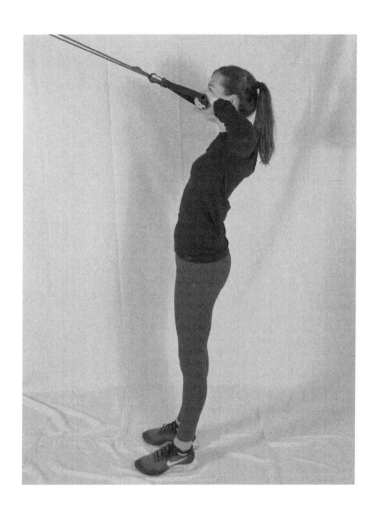

Face Pulls 2

Your lats (the latissimus dorsi muscles) are rather important in our overall functional strength. They get worked in almost all the big full-body movements described in Chapter Six, as well as many of the power movements in Chapter Seven. It is good to focus on them individually from time to time. Every commercial gym has some sort of lat pull-down machine, and depending on the attachment, you can do these with a wide or narrow grip. I recommend performing those exercises by leaning slightly back and bringing the bar down to your sternum.

If you're not in a gym, the **lat pull-down** is another exercise that can be easily performed with an exercise band. It needs to be anchored relatively high up (this one is anchored to a pull-up bar.) You simply sit or stand beneath it such that you can grasp the handles of the band with extended arms and pull it down toward you. Elizabeth could change the angle of this by sitting farther back and pulling it toward her chest as well. It is basically the vertical version of the row.

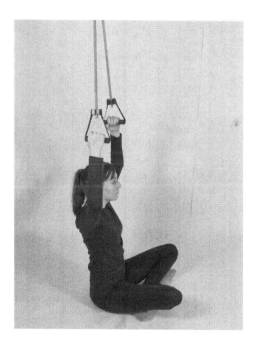

Lat Pull-downs 1

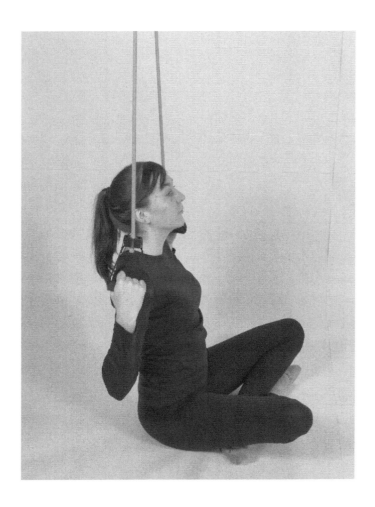

Lat Pull-downs 2

A **lat press-down** is a slightly different exercise that targets the lats in a different way. Again, the band is anchored high and with straight arms extended in front of you to hold onto the handles, you push down until your arms are in line with your torso.

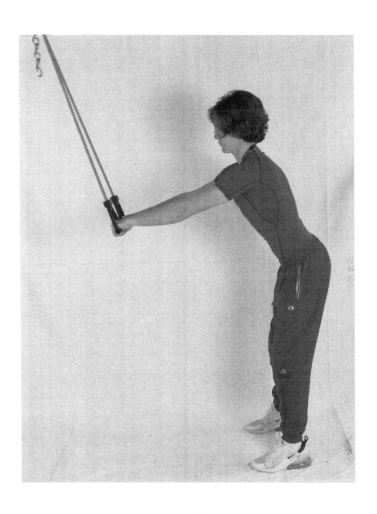

Lat Press-downs 1

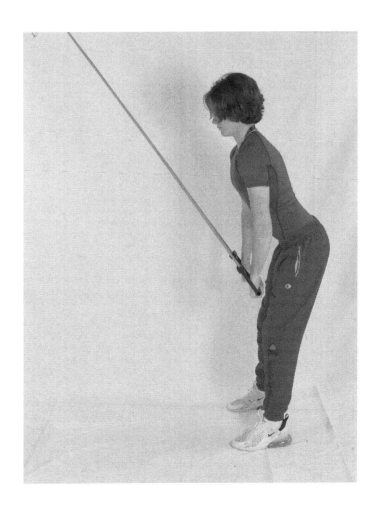

Lat Press-downs 2

If you don't have a bench, a floor press is a perfectly fine substitution. It's easier to be passive on this lift, so I would still recommend pushing your butt and upper back down into the floor to create some tension in your back. The floor limits how far back your shoulders can move, so this is a good option for people for whom the regular bench press is uncomfortable.

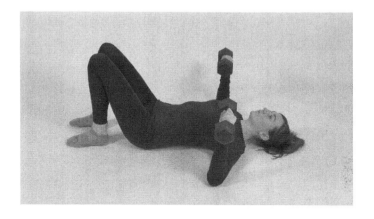

Floor Press 1

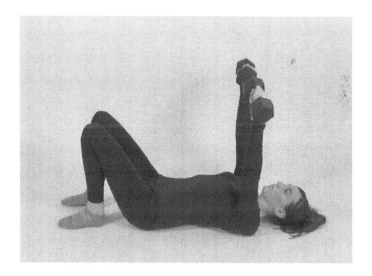

Floor Press 2

Pull-ups are basically a lat pulldown where you pull yourself up instead of pulling the weight down. There are many ways to do these and many ways to hurt yourself doing these, so let's start at the beginning. We talked about the xiphoid process in Chapter Five and how it can cause shoulder impingement. I have the kind that causes me to have pain with bar pressing, and it also affects my ability to do pull-ups with my hands pronated (facing forward). However, doing pull-ups with a pronated grip is not necessary. You can do chin-ups, with your palms facing you, or depending on your pull-up bar or attachments, you can also do pull-ups with your palms facing one another. I have found two solutions for myself, which is to either do them from rings or handles that allow me to have a neutral grip or use a mixed grip where one palm faces toward me and the other faces away.

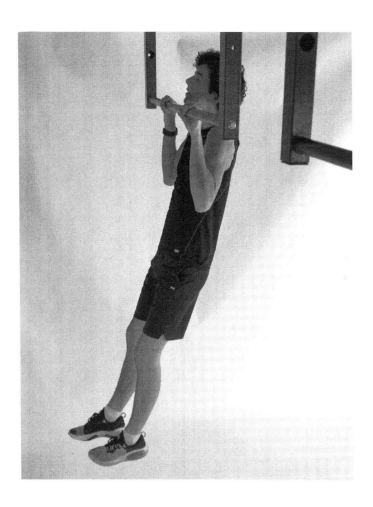

Pull-up

Now, how do we get to doing full pull-ups? Well, there are a couple of things to keep in mind. The first is that you don't have to. You can use a band to assist your body weight, or you can even keep a chair below you and give yourself a boost with your leg. You never want to be in a situation where you can't lower yourself with control from the top of the pull-up as this can excessively strain your shoulders.

When people come to me and want to be able to do a full pull-up, we start with negatives. This means that you find a way to get into the top position, arms bent, chin over bar, and you lower yourself down slowly and with control. (If you can't lower yourself with control for at least three reps, you need to spend some time getting stronger). You can jump up or use a chair to get into the top position. You don't want to do more than three to five reps of these at a time. I will have clients do three to five sets of three to five negatives at the start of their workout. Typically, they will be able to get a full pull-up within several weeks.

A **good morning** is a great exercise for strengthening your low back and hips. You can put a bar on your back as shown in the photo, or you can hold a plate or other weight in front of you close to your chest. Then you simply push your hips back and bend forward. You can keep your knees stiff or have a slight bend in them.

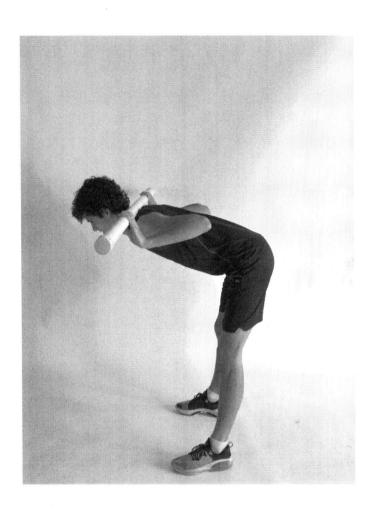

Good Morning 1

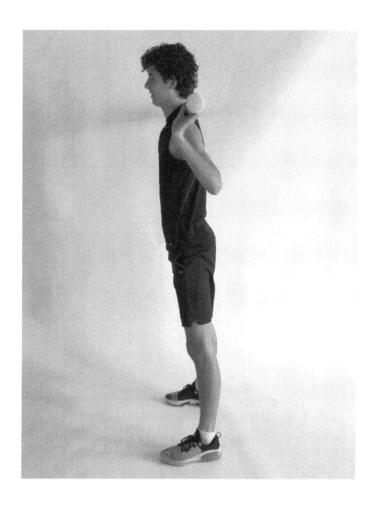

Good Morning 2

FOAM ROLLING

Foam rolling is a great way to relax tight muscles. When clients come to the gym stiff and sore from their last workout or some chronic stiffness, I have them spend about five to ten minutes rolling out all their stiff areas. You can buy one of these black Styrofoam rollers online for about $30, and they are absolutely worth it. You can also use a tennis ball to target smaller areas.

The internet is full of complicated explanations as to why or how foam rolling works. To keep it simple, you have pressure receptors in your muscles that when pressed, will respond by relaxing the muscle. This is basically how massage works. So, you want to think of this as giving yourself a massage. In the photos below, Elizabeth is rolling out her quads, her hamstrings, and her glute medius. You can target virtually any area you can reach and are only limited by what positions you can get into.

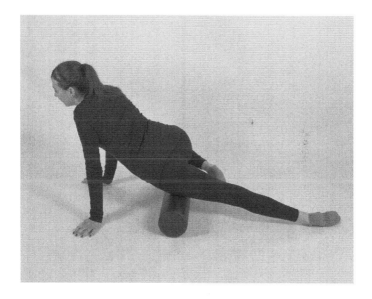

Quad Roll

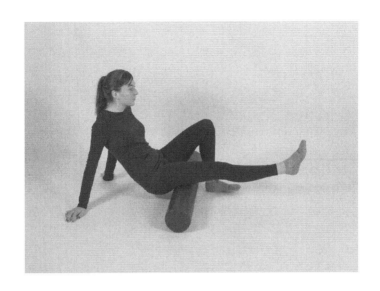

Hamstring Roll

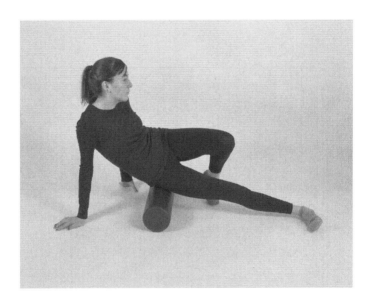

Gluteus Medius Roll

Other areas to consider are your glutes, your low back, your upper back, your shins and calves, and your IT bands (this is a thick band of connective tissue that runs down the outside of your thigh and can contribute to knee pain.) A word of warning, when you have a particularly tight muscle, foam rolling can be rather painful. If you aren't sure if a muscle is injured or just tight, it is probably a good idea to reach out to your doctor.

APPENDIX B

EVOLUTION AND WHY DIET IS IMPORTANT

In Chapter Four, we briefly talked about Herman Pontzer's work on the health of modern hunter-gatherer societies. One aspect I mentioned and did not elaborate on was his findings on daily calorie expenditure of these societies as compared to Western societies. What his research has shown is that relative to lean body mass and age, the total energy expenditure of these individuals is not very different from Westerners with either active or sedentary lifestyles. This means that the average sedentary American and your average gym-going American both burn about the same number of calories as your average hunter-gatherer.[135]

That last bit may have perked your ears up a little, and quite honestly, it kind of blew my mind a bit as well. In another comprehensive review article on the energy expenditure of

---

135   H. Pontzer, B. M. Wood, and D. A. Raichlen, "Hunter-Gatherers as Models in Public Health," *Obesity Reviews* 19, no. S1 (December 1, 2018): 24–30.

primates, Pontzer demonstrated that this *constrained total energy expenditure is species-specific with a definitive upper limit regardless of additional physical activity.*[136]

I highlighted that last statement because I realize it's complicated. What it means in layman's terms is that regardless of how much exercise you get, there is a limit as to how many calories you can burn in a day. This means we have to control our calorie intake if we want to control our weight.

To summarize what we learned in Chapter Four, we evolved to walk upright and have big brains. These two things allowed us to navigate and travel long distances to hunt and gather food. We store fat more easily than other primates to prevent starvation on our long journeys. Another survival advantage was the complexity of our societies, which allowed for task and food sharing. Our brains and bodies are intrinsically linked to perform those tasks. Without those tasks, our bodies and our brains do not function optimally.

The crux of that research is that we require physical activity for physical health, brain health, and optimal cognitive function. It is not, however, the most effective way to decrease excess body fat, which is important for our overall health. Although physical activity does help improve health markers in the overweight, it is not to the same degree that occurs in individuals with healthier weight. Physical activity *and* fat

---

136 Herman Pontzer, "The Crown Joules: Energetics, Ecology, and Evolution in Humans and Other Primates," *Evolutionary Anthropology: Issues, News, and Reviews* 26, no. 1 (January 1, 2017): 16–17.

loss are optimal for reducing disease and joint damage.[137] Excess weight can cause a number of orthopedic issues that affect the spine, shoulders, knees, feet, wrists, and ankles. These include osteoarthritis, chronic pain, and a greater risk of injury.[138] Joint pain also prevents us from being more physically active, which in turn decreases our resistance to disease.

For the record, I do not advocate the notion that everyone needs to walk around with six-pack abs or look like a fitness competitor. Those levels of body fat are not particularly healthy either, especially for women. As I stated at the end of Chapter Three, you can use BMI or waist circumference to determine if you are at a healthy weight.

WHY DOESN'T INCREASING OUR PHYSICAL ACTIVITY SIGNIFICANTLY INCREASE THE NUMBER OF CALORIES WE BURN?

Our bodies *do* increase daily energy expenditure (DEE) with exercise, and the fitter you are, the higher your DEE is likely to be…to a point. Our bodies are masters at adapting to stress, and one of the ways we adapt to regular exercise is to become more fuel efficient, i.e., over time, we will burn fewer calories for the same amount of activity. This happens in a couple of ways:

---

137 Pedro L. Valenzuela et al., "Joint Association of Physical Activity and Body Mass Index with Cardiovascular Risk: A Nationwide Population-Based Cross-Sectional Study," *European Journal of Preventive Cardiology*, no. zwaa151 (January 22, 2021).

138 Harvard Health Publishing, "Why Weight Matters When It Comes to Joint Pain," *Harvard Health*.

1. Our bodies get better at burning fat for fuel rather than sugar, which makes us more fuel efficient. Fat contains more than twice the calories per gram than sugar, so relying on fat-burning pathways actually slows down how much fuel we use. For example, it has been shown in runners that energy expenditure increases to a certain point when they begin training. After several weeks, this energy expenditure plateaus and does not increase despite large increases in daily activity.[139]
2. Introducing a moderate to vigorous exercise routine to individuals often results in them being less active in other parts of their day. They sit more and move less overall, whether it be not getting up as often or simply not fidgeting as much. In other words, they rest more to make up for the energy they just expended.[140]
3. At higher levels of activity, our bodies may begin to shunt calories during exercise away from non-muscular functions such as hormone production, immune system activities, and other maintenance activities.[141]

This upper limit on energy expenditure in humans regardless of activity level is important in that less than half of the energy we expend is due to physical activity. The majority of the calories we burn are spent on our body's basic operation

139 Klaas R. Westerterp, "Exercise, Energy Balance and Body Composition," *European Journal of Clinical Nutrition* 72, no. 9 (September 2018): 1247.

140 K. R. Westerterp, "Control of Energy Expenditure in Humans," *European Journal of Clinical Nutrition* 71, no. 3 (March 1, 2017): 340–3.; Pontzer, "The Crown Joules: Energetics, Ecology, and Evolution in Humans and Other Primates,": 18.

141 Herman Pontzer et al., "Constrained Total Energy Expenditure and Metabolic Adaptation to Physical Activity in Adult Humans," *Current Biology : CB* 26, no. 3 (February 8, 2016): 414.

and maintenance activities.[142] The less healthy we are, the more maintenance we require. Instead of having energy available for fighting off infections and moving more, energy is mostly spent on things an otherwise healthy body doesn't need. In order to be optimally healthy, we have to move.

"Our bodies are evolved to require daily physical activity, and consequently, exercise does not make our bodies work more so much as it makes them work better.... Instead, exercise regulates the way the body spends energy and coordinates vital tasks."

HERMAN PONTZER[143]

Beyond a certain point, no matter how many additional calories you add, how much sleep you get, or how well-trained you are, excess exercise will result in overtraining syndrome, a rather serious condition that results in chronic fatigue, depression, and damage to the nervous system and immune function. This typically happens in high-level athletes, though it can happen in anyone with a physically demanding job. What is happening here is that the level of activity the individual is engaging in requires more calories

---

142 Westerterp, "Control of Energy Expenditure in Humans,": 340–3.

143 Herman Pontzer, "Evolved to Exercise," *Scientific American*, January 2019: 29.

than your body is willing to part with, and as a result, it begins to shut down.[144]

On the other end of the spectrum, how do we account for a relatively high daily energy expenditure in heavier-set, more sedentary individuals?

This one is a bit easier to answer, and you can think of this as the antithesis of the overtrained elite athlete. In individuals with higher body fat percentages, regular activities are much more physically taxing, so they are performed less often and with more rest in between efforts.[145] And it's not surprising; imagine how difficult it would be to do all your daily activities with an extra hundred pounds or two strapped to your back. Additionally, larger bodies not only require more calories for basic movement, but they also require more physiological maintenance and repair than average individuals, which accounts for a large portion of the calories burned.[146] Like the overtrained athlete, there is a limit on how energy can be spent on repair and maintenance.

We simply cannot choose diet OR exercise; they both play important, but separate roles in our health and body composition.

---

144 Jeffrey B. Kreher and Jennifer B. Schwartz, "Overtraining Syndrome: A Practical Guide," *Sports Health* 4, no. 2 (March 2012): 128–37.; Pontzer, "The Crown Joules: Energetics, Ecology, and Evolution in Humans and Other Primates,": 18–9.

145 Westerterp, "Exercise, Energy Balance and Body Composition,": 1248.

146 Westerterp, "Control of Energy Expenditure in Humans,": 340–3.

WHAT IS IMPORTANT TO KNOW ABOUT DIET

Many people have different thoughts about how many calories, carbohydrates, fats, and protein we need each day, and it's hard to sift through all the information and come up with an exact number. Even though traditional hunter-gatherer lifestyles are associated with good health and lower body fat, their diets are extremely varied, so it is difficult to glean any conclusions about what an ideal human diet may be. The only commonalities seem to be that most humans eat a mixture of plants and animals and cook their food.[147]

It gets even more complicated than that. When we eat, we are feeding both our bodies and our gut bacteria. Gut bacteria have been implicated in excess body fat accumulation, and this finding seems to be based on both the type of bacteria and what the bacteria is feeding on. Optimizing nutrients for both our own unique selves and the microorganisms in our gut is never going to be a cut and dried exact prescription.[148] The truth is, nutritional research is still in its infancy, so be wary of anyone telling you that a certain macro-nutrient ratio is the gold standard for everyone. They are wrong.

Finding the ideal diet for you and your lifestyle is going to require some observation and practice. You need to start by having a realistic understanding of portion sizes and

---

147 Pontzer, Wood, and Raichlen, "Hunter-Gatherers as Models in Public Health,": 31.

148 Louise Crovesy, Daniele Masterson, and Eliane Lopes Rosado, "Profile of the Gut Microbiota of Adults with Obesity: A Systematic Review," *European Journal of Clinical Nutrition* 74, no. 9 (September 1, 2020): 1251.; François Leulier et al., "Integrative Physiology: At the Crossroads of Nutrition, Microbiota, Animal Physiology, and Human Health," *Cell Metabolism* 25, no. 3 (March 7, 2017): 527–30.

nutrition facts. These figures are readily available on all food packaging, in a number of books, websites, and food tracking apps you can download to your phone. Tracking your diet is not something you necessarily have to commit to for a lifetime. It is, however, something you should learn to do. Tracking your diet even for a couple of months will give you a much better idea as to how many calories you are consuming each day as well as how many grams of carbohydrates, fats, and protein.

DAILY CALORIE RECOMMENDATIONS ARE JUST A STARTING POINT

It is important that you understand that when you do an initial calculation to determine your caloric needs that this is just a starting point. Everyone is different and will require different numbers of calories depending on their unique genetics and daily activity. That being said, there isn't a great deal of variation. The quality of your food will make a big difference in how much volume you can eat and how many nutrients you will get out of your food. For example, a Snickers bar only has seventy fewer calories than a grilled chicken sandwich on a whole grain roll with honey mustard, lettuce, and tomato. That chicken sandwich has way more protein and nutrients. I'm not saying you can't have a Snickers bar, just that if you do, it just took a big chunk out of your daily calorie requirement without supplying many essential nutrients. Choose your foods wisely.

If you need a starting number, most adult women need between 1,800 and 2,400 calories a day. Most adult men need between 2,200 and 2,800 calories a day. These numbers range from sedentary to very active lifestyles and will also have some variation based on body size, age, and genetics. Regardless, as you can see, they aren't very different, so start tracking what you are eating and make conservative changes as you go. For more information, check out the FDA resource, myplate.gov.[149]

PROTEIN

The number one nutrient that most people are deficient in is protein. It used to be thought that high protein diets were bad, especially for older adults. It was erroneously thought that high protein diets would cause bone loss or kidney problems. This is not true.[150] Older adults are actually at risk of losing muscle as they age, and as we talked about in Chapter Five, this muscle loss, sarcopenia, is associated with early death. A higher protein diet in combination with resistance training has been shown to prevent and reverse sarcopenia in elderly patients.[151] Higher protein diets are also thought to prevent or slow the progress of dementia and Alzheimer's as well.[152]

It must be noted here that the quality of the protein matters. A diet high in saturated fats, sugars, and processed foods will not benefit your health regardless of how much protein you

---

149 "MyPlate," US Department of Agriculture."

150 Denise Webb, "Protein for Fitness: Age Demands Greater Protein Needs," *Today's Dietician*, April 2015.

151 Hidekatsu Yanai, "Nutrition for Sarcopenia," *Journal of Clinical Medicine Research* 7, no. 12 (December 2015): 926–30.

152 Jordan M. Glenn, Erica N. Madero, and Nick T Bott, "Dietary Protein and Amino Acid Intake: Links to the Maintenance of Cognitive Health," *Nutrients* 11, no. 6, article no. 1315 (June 12, 2019).

are eating. Fish, poultry, lean cuts of meat, legumes, whole grains, and lean dairy are all good sources of protein.

CARBOHYDRATES AND FAT

Carbohydrates and fats are energy calories that also play a vital role in our bodies' structure and function. Carbohydrates contain four calories per gram, like protein, while fats contain nine calories per gram. The ratio of fat to carbohydrate calories in your diet is something that should be optimized by your own observations. Personally, I stick to a higher carbohydrate to fat ratio for both energy and body composition. I know others who do the opposite. My typical ratios are about 30 percent protein, 30 percent fat, and 40 percent carbohydrates. That varies depending on my goals and how much attention I'm willing to pay.

Fat is a very important part of your nervous system, hormones, and cell membranes and acts as carrier molecules for fat-soluble vitamins and other important nutrients. As with protein, the quality of fats in your diet is very important. Although we do need some saturated fats in our diet, diets high in saturated fats and processed foods are more likely to cause a host of health problems. Stick to nuts, seeds, olive oil, lean meats and fish, and avocados whenever possible.[153]

Carbohydrates are an essential fuel source, especially for our brains. Carbohydrates help us grow and maintain our muscle mass and dietary fiber is great for the health of our digestive tract. In fact, dietary fiber can help reduce our blood

---

153 Harvard Health Publishing, "Know the Facts about Fats," *Harvard Health*.

cholesterol by absorbing and eliminating bile, which would otherwise be resorbed and has been associated with good heart health. As with protein and fats, quality is incredibly important. Try to choose foods that are high in fiber and low in added sugar.[154]

WHY WE OVER-EAT AND WHY IT'S NOT NECESSARILY OUR FAULT

In *The Third Plate*, Dan Barber explores the development of sustainable agriculture that results in both flavorful and nutrient-rich foods. One of the anecdotes he tells in the first few chapters explains how soil quality will play a leading role in developing superior plants and livestock. Simply put, it's been shown that cattle grazing on land with nutrient-enriched soil consume less grass than cattle grazing on land with nutrient-depleted soil. They overeat the less nutritious food in an effort to satisfy their requirement of essential nutrients. When their food is nutritionally dense, they eat less.[155] How do they know which grass is more nutritious? It may all come down to flavor.

In "The Dorito Effect," journalist Mark Schatzker reviews how food and food science has changed in the last several decades. It has changed how we grow crops, feed livestock, and create unnatural flavors to mask the bland flavors of mass-produced, less nutritious food. Ultimately, taste is supposed to signal to us what nutrients are contained in the food,

---

154 "What Are the Key Functions of Carbohydrates?" Healthline, November 9, 2017.

155 Dan Barber, *The Third Plate : Field Notes on the Future of Food* (New York: The Penguin Press, 2014): 97–99.

and our brains then learn to crave different flavors based on our needs.

Unfortunately, our farming practices in the last century have focused on appearance, size, and pest resistance, not necessarily flavor. Mass produced foods have become deficient in flavor and compounds that are necessary for our health. They are also deficient in the compounds that send a signal to our body when we've had "enough." Instead of fixing the "bland" problem by raising more high-quality foods, artificial flavoring has become the solution for the food industry.[156]

Artificial flavors falsely indicate nutrients that aren't present, which makes us want to eat more. Processed and artificially flavored foods do not contain the nutrients and secondary compounds that would signal that we've had enough. There is a saying that the only difference between medicine and poison is the dose. When feeding naturally, animals seem to be able to discern exactly how much of a certain plant (or animal) they need to eat to benefit them with overdosing. Sheep have been known to eat baby birds when they are mineral deficient. However, livestock can also be fooled with artificial flavors. An additive called Sucram is routinely used to increase feeding volume of normally unpalatable foods and get younger animals on solid foods sooner.[157]

What are these "secondary compounds" that signal us to limit consumption? Plants have naturally occurring compounds

---

156 Mark Schatzker, *The Dorito Effect: The Surprising New Truth About Food and Flavor* (New York: Simon and Schuster Paperbacks, 2015): 19–40.

157 Ibid., 109–134.

that protect them from being consumed. In small amounts, these compounds are benign and even beneficial to our health. If the dose is too high, they may be harmful. When we have consumed the maximum useful amount of these compounds, our bodies tell us to stop. The problem with processed foods is that even though they may contain some of these compounds, they don't contain enough to limit our consumption to a healthy level. The same company that developed Sucram to promote overfeeding discovered that when using oregano extract for intestinal health in pigs, too high a dose limited how much feed the pigs would eat.[158]

I want you to think about the times you have eaten to the point of discomfort as compared to the times you felt satisfied and not interested in eating any more. What kinds of foods left you feeling satisfied without feeling uncomfortable?

CHANGING YOUR DIET BEHAVIOR
When I counsel clients on fat loss, I try to take a strategic approach rather than a strict prescription. I feel that most people benefit more from changes in habits and behaviors rather than trying to stick to a rigidly prescribed set of numbers. Rigid prescriptions work for some and are essential if you ever want to compete in a bodybuilding or figure competition. However, speaking from personal experience, that approach can be complicated and stressful. Below are the behaviors that I encourage everyone to adopt over time, and the very first one is the most important.

---

158 Ibid., 149–157.

KEEP A DIET JOURNAL

Online apps make tracking your diet very easy to do these days. The most important part about keeping a journal is that it allows us to see what works and what doesn't work. Keeping a realistic account of your diet, your training schedule, and general sense of well-being is extremely important to your success. If you are honest with yourself regarding what and how much you eat, you may see some areas you can improve right away. For example, maybe that morning latte has way too much sugar or what you thought was one serving of rice was actually three. That being said, don't try and make too many changes too soon. Very few people can make a drastic change in their diet and stick to it for the long term.

PROTEIN FIRST AND WITH EVERY MEAL

For too long our American diet fads have focused on reducing fat or carbohydrates. However, the key macronutrient that will determine our success in terms of building and repairing muscle and connective tissue, supporting immune function, and synthesizing essential biomolecules such as enzymes and hormones is protein.

Most people don't get enough protein.

The first change we need to make in our diets is to make sure that we are getting our daily protein requirement, roughly one to one-and-a-half grams per kg of body weight daily.[159]

---

159 Nancy R. Rodriguez, "Introduction to Protein Summit 2.0: Continued Exploration of the Impact of High-Quality Protein on Optimal Health," *The American Journal of Clinical Nutrition* 101, no. 6 (June 1, 2015): 1317S–1319S.

For an individual weighing 165 pounds (75 kg), that is a range of 75–113 grams of protein per day.

Prioritizing lean protein sources will automatically change the character of your meals by adding more whole grains, lean meats, and protein-rich vegetables such as legumes.

KEEP PROCESSED FOODS TO A MINIMUM
All refined and processed foods are broken down very quickly in the gut. In the case of refined flours and sugars, this means that they get into the bloodstream very quickly and efficiently, which delivers a huge load of calories that we don't really need. These are also devoid of fiber, protein, and micronutrients that are usually found in real food.

Processed foods often contain fats not found in nature such as partially hydrogenated vegetable oils (trans fats). These fats have been associated with an increased risk of cardiovascular disease.[160]

Eat more real food. Keep a ready supply of fruit and vegetables in your house or on your office desk. Cook at home as often as possible.

MEAL TIMING IS OF THE UTMOST IMPORTANCE
The research on frequency and timing of meals indicates that eating the bulk of your calories earlier in the day is more beneficial for both health and weight loss. Consuming the

---

160 "Trans Fat: Double Trouble for Your Heart," Mayo Clinic.

bulk of your calories later in the day rather than earlier is associated with higher cardiovascular disease risk and weight gain.[161] For those who have an odd schedule or do shift work, think about consuming the bulk of your calories during the most active times of your day.

MEAL PREP

The hardest thing about eating well is giving up convenience foods. Our lives are busy, hectic, and sometimes just completely crazy. Getting a cheeseburger at the drive-thru may seem easier than preparing a whole food meal from scratch. Instead, it is relatively easy to make a big batch of stew, a casserole, or even a batch of grilled meat that you can pack into individual containers and use for several days. However, if your lifestyle makes meal prepping difficult, do your research. Most restaurants, including fast food restaurants, post their nutrition information online. Educate yourself and make better choices.

DON'T STARVE YOURSELF

I have seen far too many individuals sacrifice energy, overall health, and even bone density in the quest for "skinny." You will look and feel far better if you build a strong body first; any extra pounds will be much easier to shed with metabolically active muscle to help burn it off. On a healthy diet,

---

161 M. Garaulet et al., "Timing of Food Intake Predicts Weight Loss Effectiveness," *International Journal of Obesity* 37, no. 4 (April 1, 2013): 606–10.; Antonio Paoli et al., "The Influence of Meal Frequency and Timing on Health in Humans: The Role of Fasting," *Nutrients* 11, no. 4 (March 28, 2019): 719.

after the initial adjustment period, you should NOT feel tired, run-down, depressed, injured, or unmotivated. This can be a sign that you are missing critical nutrients or simply not getting enough calories. Making small adjustments works far better than drastic changes.

TRACK YOUR PROGRESS

Using a scale is fine. To measure more subtle changes in body composition that aren't reflected in scale weight, use tape measurements of your waist, hips, thighs, arms, and neck to track progress. Oftentimes the number on the scale will go up when you first begin an exercise program due to increased muscle mass and bone density. The tape measure or simply a weekly selfie in your underwear can show you progress when the scale isn't moving much.

***

The bottom line here is that exercise is just not as direct a route to fat loss as diet. Strength training and aerobic training change our bodies in ways that makes us healthier, more resistant to disease, and able to do more things. Diet, however, is the most direct and more important way to reduce body fat over time. Do not make the mistake of choosing only one, you need both movement and a healthy diet to be as healthy and fit as possible.

ACKNOWLEDGMENTS

I would like to sincerely thank those who backed this project, sight unseen, while I was still in the writing process. I appreciate your faith, your feedback, and your curiosity.

Alexandra Duncan

Allison Snead

Allys Dierker

Amy Jenkins

Amy Spyker

Aslynn Halvorson

Brandon Cooke

Cheri Wissmann

Chris McClinch

Christina Cash

Christine Bjerke

Christopher Parker

Cindy Lehman

Coya Bird

Deann Arbutina

Deanna Sohn

Elijah smith

Emmanuel Robinson

Eric Koester

Frank Fleming

Frankie Winn

Gail Hemedinger

Gant Grimes

Gregory Adams

Ingrid Marcum

James Budinetz

Jeremy Rusnock

Jerold Rusnock

Justine Crowley

Karina Rodriguez

Kristine Kobza

Lloyd Jenkins

Lynn Yap

Mark Saye

Mark Sullivan

Maureen Petron

Mereth Alexander

Michael Fleming

Michele Murdock

Michelle Karten

Mike McAloon

Myriah Velazco

Patricia Debnam

Patricia Fleming

Patrick Hammond

Paul Lussier

Penny Crittenden

Rachel Barrett

Renee Croteau

Luke Neu

Rita McDonnell

Roman Placzek

Sandy Thompson

Stacey Torres

Stacye Bruckbauer

Stan Barrett

Stephen Saks

Steve Hollosi

Tanya Parise

Stephanie Jenny

Tiffany Anderson

Tim Keutzer

Valerie MacNabb

Vicky Lehman

I would also like to thank my friends and colleagues who spent time listening to and discussing my ideas, reading rough drafts, and sharing their thoughts on this project. I value your insight and expertise, and your input helped shape the depth and direction of this book. Sal Aria, Tom Furman, Alex Hoffman, Justin Keane, Mike McKenna, Gregory Morris, and Bethany Wadsworth, I am grateful for your thoughts and your time.

A big thank you to my photo models Elizabeth Fleming, Francis Fleming, Patrick Fleming, Shani Inbari, and Laura Marston. This book would require a lot more imagination without you.

Most importantly, I would like to thank Eric Koester for the opportunity to create this book. I could not have done this without my editors, Kyrsten Rice and Bianca DaSilva, as well as the rest of the team at New Degree Press.

You all have my deepest gratitude.

BIBLIOGRAPHY

INTRODUCTION

Aicale, R., D. Tarantino, and N. Maffulli. "Overuse Injuries in Sport: A Comprehensive Overview." *Journal of Orthopaedic Surgery and Research* 13, no. 1, article no. 309 (December 5, 2018): 1–11. *https://doi.org/10.1186/s13018-018-1017-5.*

Lachman, Margie E., Lewis Lipsitz, James Lubben, Carmen Casta-neda-Sceppa, and Alan M. Jette. "When Adults Don't Exercise: Behavioral Strategies to Increase Physical Activity in Sedentary Middle-Aged and Older Adults." *Innovation in Aging* 2, no. igy007 (April 5, 2018). *https://doi.org/10.1093/geroni/igy007.*

Lee, Harold H., Jessica A. Emerson, and David M. Williams. "The Exercise–Affect–Adherence Pathway: An Evolutionary Perspective." *Frontiers in Psychology* 7, article no. 1285 (2016): 1–11. *https://doi.org/10.3389/fpsyg.2016.01285.*

Pontzer, Herman. "The Crown Joules: Energetics, Ecology, and Evolution in Humans and Other Primates." *Evolutionary Anthropology: Issues, News, and Reviews* 26, no. 1 (January 1, 2017): 12–24. *https://doi.org/10.1002/evan.21513.*

Powell, Kenneth E., Amanda E. Paluch, and Steven N. Blair. "Physical Activity for Health: What Kind? How Much? How Intense? On Top of What?" *Annual Review of Public Health* 32, no. 1 (March 18, 2011): 349–65. *https://doi.org/10.1146/annurev-publhealth-031210-101151.*

Rutgers University. "High-Intensity Interval Training Increases Injuries, Research Shows: White Men Aged 20 to 39 Were Injured Most, Study Finds." ScienceDaily press release, April 9, 2019. Accessed January 15, 2021. *www.sciencedaily.com/releases/2019/04/190409083239.htm.*

Seiler, Stephen. "How 'Normal People' Can Train like the World's Best Endurance Athletes." Filmed November 2019 in Arendal, Norway. *TEDx Talk,* 16:04. *https://www.ted.com/talks/stephen_seiler_how_normal_people_can_train_like_the_worlds_best_edurance_athletes.*

Seiler, Stephen, and Espen Tonnessen. "Intervals, Thresholds, and Long Slow Distance: The Role of Intensity and Duration in Endurance Training." *Sports Science* 13 (2009): 32–53. sportsci.org/2009/ss.htm.

Verkhoshansky, Yuri, and Mel C. Siff. *Supertraining.* Sixth Edition-Expanded Version. Rome: Verkoshansky, 2009.

CHAPTER 1

Carini, Francesco, Margherita Mazzola, Chiara Fici, Salvatore Palmeri, Massimo Messina, Provvidenza Damiani, and Giovanni Tomasello. "Posture and Posturology, Anatomical and Physiological Profiles: Overview and Current State of Art." *Acta Bio-Medica : Atenei Parmensis* 88, no. 1 (April 28, 2017): 11–16. *https://doi.org/10.23750/abm.v88i1.5309.*

Cunha, Carolina Ortigosa, Lívia Maria Sales Pinto-Fiamengui, Fernanda Araújo Sampaio, and Paulo César Rodrigues Conti.

"Is Aerobic Exercise Useful to Manage Chronic Pain?" *Revista Dor* 17 (2016): 61–64.

Dahab, Katherine Stabenow, and Teri Metcalf McCambridge. "Strength Training in Children and Adolescents: Raising the Bar for Young Athletes?" *Sports Health* 1, no.3 (May 2009): 223–26. *https://doi.org/10.1177/1941738109334215.*

Hatfield, Frederick. *Fitness: The Complete Guide.* 9th ed. Carpinteria, CA: International Sports Sciences Association, 2018.

Kato, Satoshi, Hideki Murakami, Satoru Demura, Katsuhito Yoshioka, Kazuya Shinmura, Noriaki Yokogawa, Takashi Igarashi, Noritaka Yonezawa, Takaki Shimizu, and Hiroyuki Tsuchiya. "Abdominal Trunk Muscle Weakness and Its Association with Chronic Low Back Pain and Risk of Falling in Older Women." *BMC Musculoskeletal Disorders* 20, no. 1 (June 3, 2019): 273–273. *https://doi.org/10.1186/s12891-019-2655-4.*

Kim, DeokJu, MiLim Cho, YunHee Park, and YeongAe Yang. "Effect of an Exercise Program for Posture Correction on Musculoskeletal Pain." *Journal of Physical Therapy Science* 27, no. 6 (June 2015): 1791–94. *https://doi.org/10.1589/jpts.27.1791.*

Kwak, Seong-Eun, Ji-Hyun Lee, Didi Zhang, and Wook Song. "Angiogenesis: Focusing on the Effects of Exercise in Aging and Cancer." *Journal of Exercise Nutrition & Biochemistry* 22, no. 3 (September 30, 2018): 21–26. *https://doi.org/10.20463/jenb.2018.0020.*

Lachman, Margie E., Lewis Lipsitz, James Lubben, Carmen Castaneda-Sceppa, and Alan M. Jette. "When Adults Don't Exercise: Behavioral Strategies to Increase Physical Activity in Sedentary Middle-Aged and Older Adults." *Innovation in Aging* 2, no. igy007 (April 5, 2018). *https://doi.org/10.1093/geroni/igy007.*

Lee, Harold H., Jessica A. Emerson, and David M. Williams. "The Exercise–Affect–Adherence Pathway: An Evolutionary Perspective." *Frontiers in Psychology* 7, article no. 1285 (2016): 1–11. *https://doi.org/10.3389/fpsyg.2016.01285.*

McLeod, Michael, Leigh Breen, D. Lee Hamilton, and Andrew Philp. "Live Strong and Prosper: The Importance of Skeletal Muscle Strength for Healthy Ageing." *Biogerontology* 17, no. 3 (June 2016): 497–510. *https://doi.org/10.1007/s10522-015-9631-7.*

Nystoriak, Matthew A., and Aruni Bhatnagar. "Cardiovascular Effects and Benefits of Exercise." *Frontiers in Cardiovascular Medicine* 5 (September 28, 2018): 135–135. *https://doi.org/10.3389/fcvm.2018.00135.*

O'Keefe JH Jr and Cordain L. "Cardiovascular Disease Resulting from a Diet and Lifestyle at Odds with Our Paleolithic Genome: How to Become a 21st-Century Hunter-Gatherer." *Mayo Clinic Proceedings* 79, no. 1 (2004): 101–8.

Olfert, I Mark, Oliver Baum, Ylva Hellsten, and Stuart Egginton. "Advances and Challenges in Skeletal Muscle Angiogenesis." *American Journal of Physiology. Heart and Circulatory Physiology* 310, no. 3 (February 1, 2016): H326–36. *https://doi.org/10.1152/ajpheart.00635.2015.*

O'Mara, Shane. *In Praise of Walking: The New Science of How We Walk and Why It's Good for Us.* New York: W. W. Norton & Company, 2020. (book)

US Department of Health and Human Services. Physical Activity Guidelines for Americans, 2nd edition. Washington, DC: US Department of Health and Human Services; 2018. *https://health.gov/sites/default/files/2019-09/Physical_Activity_Guidelines_2nd_edition.pdf*

Pontzer, Herman. "The Crown Joules: Energetics, Ecology, and Evolution in Humans and Other Primates." *Evolutionary Anthropology: Issues, News, and Reviews* 26, no. 1 (January 1, 2017): 12–24. *https://doi.org/10.1002/evan.21513.*

Powell, Kenneth E., Amanda E. Paluch, and Steven N. Blair. "Physical Activity for Health: What Kind? How Much? How Intense? On Top of What?" *Annual Review of Public Health* 32, no. 1 (March 18, 2011): 349–65. *https://doi.org/10.1146/annurev-publhealth-031210-101151.*

Rosa, João P. P., Altay A. L. de Souza, Giscard H. O. de Lima, Dayane F. Rodrigues, Valdir de Aquino Lemos, Eduardo da Silva Alves, Sergio Tufik, and Marco T. de Mello. "Motivational and Evolutionary Aspects of a Physical Exercise Training Program: A Longitudinal Study." *Frontiers in Psychology* 6 (May 18, 2015): 648–648. *https://doi.org/10.3389/fpsyg.2015.00648.*

Sale, Digby G. "Neural Adaptation to Resistance Training." *Medicine & Science in Sports & Exercise* 20, no. 5 (1988): S135–S145. *https://journals.lww.com/acsm-msse/Fulltext/1988/10001/Neural_adaptation_to_resistance_training.9.aspx.*

"Strength Training by Children and Adolescents." *Pediatrics* 121, no. 4 (April 1, 2008): 835–840. *https://doi.org/10.1542/peds.2007-3790.*

Verkhoshansky, Yuri, and Mel C. Siff. *Supertraining.* Sixth Edition-Expanded Version. Rome: Verkoshansky, 2009.

CHAPTER 2

Aicale, R., D. Tarantino, and N. Maffulli. "Overuse Injuries in Sport: A Comprehensive Overview." *Journal of Orthopaedic Surgery and Research* 13, no. 1, article no. 309 (December 5, 2018): 1–11. *https://doi.org/10.1186/s13018-018-1017-5.*

Gambetta, Vern, and Stephen Seiler. "GAINcast Episode 104: Polarized Training (with Stephen Seiler)." February 15, 2018 In _ Gaincast with Vern Gambetta _ produced by Vern Gambetta, podcast, MP3 audio, 56:18. *http://www.hmmrmedia. com/2018/02/gaincast-episode-104-polarized-training-with-stephen-seiler/*.

Lauersen, Jeppe Bo, Thor Einar Andersen, and Lars Bo Andersen. "Strength Training as Superior, Dose-Dependent and Safe Prevention of Acute and Overuse Sports Injuries: A Systematic Review, Qualitative Analysis and Meta-Analysis." *British Journal of Sports Medicine* 52, no. 24 (December 1, 2018): 1557–63. *https://doi.org/10.1136/bjsports-2018-099078*.

Rattray, Ben, Christos Argus, Kristy Martin, Joseph Northey, and Matthew Driller. "Is It Time to Turn Our Attention toward Central Mechanisms for Post-Exertional Recovery Strategies and Performance?" *Frontiers in Physiology* 6, article no. 79 (March 17, 2015): 1–14. *https://doi.org/10.3389/fphys.2015.00079*.

Rutgers University. "High-intensity interval training increases injuries, research shows: White men aged 20 to 39 were injured most, study finds." ScienceDaily. press release, April 9, 2019. *www.sciencedaily.com/releases/2019/04/190409083239.htm* (accessed January 15, 2021).

Seiler, Stephen. "How 'Normal People' Can Train like the World's Best Endurance Athletes." Filmed November 2019 in Arendal, Norway. *TEDx Talk, https://www.ted.com/talks/stephen_seiler_ how_normal_people_can_train_like_the_worlds_best_endurance_athletes*.

Seiler, Stephen, and Espen Tonnessen. "Intervals, Thresholds, and Long Slow Distance: The Role of Intensity and Duration in Endurance Training." *Sports Science* 13 (2009): 32–53. *sportsci. org/2009/ss.htm*.

Taylor, Janet L, Markus Amann, Jacques Duchateau, Romain Meeusen, and Charles L Rice. "Neural Contributions to Muscle Fatigue: From the Brain to the Muscle and Back Again." *Medicine and Science in Sports and Exercise* 48, no. 11 (November 2016): 2294–2306. *https://doi.org/10.1249/MSS.0000000000000923.*

Thompson, Walter R. "Worldwide Survey of Fitness Trends for 2018: The CREP Edition." *ACSM's Health & Fitness Journal* 21, no. 6 (2017): 10–19. *https://journals.lww.com/acsm-healthfitness/Fulltext/2017/11000/WORLDWIDE_SURVEY_OF_FITNESS_TRENDS_FOR_2018__The.6.aspx.*

CHAPTER 3

Andrade, Alexandro, Ricardo de Azevedo Klumb Steffens, Sofia Mendes Sieczkowska, Leonardo Alexandre Peyré Tartaruga, and Guilherme Torres Vilarino. "A Systematic Review of the Effects of Strength Training in Patients with Fibromyalgia: Clinical Outcomes and Design Considerations." *Advances in Rheumatology* 58, no. 1 (October 22, 2018): 36. *https://doi.org/10.1186/s42358-018-0033-9.*

Berry, Meredith S., Meredith A. Repke, Alexander L. Metcalf, and Kerry E. Jordan. "Promoting Healthy Decision-Making via Natural Environment Exposure: Initial Evidence and Future Directions." *Frontiers in Psychology* 11: 1682 (July 14, 2020): 1–6. *https://doi.org/10.3389/fpsyg.2020.01682.*

Bertisch, Suzanne M., Benjamin D. Pollock, Murray A. Mittleman, Daniel J. Buysse, Lydia A. Bazzano, Daniel J. Gottlieb, and Susan Redline. "Insomnia with Objective Short Sleep Duration and Risk of Incident Cardiovascular Disease and All-Cause Mortality: Sleep Heart Health Study." *Sleep* 41, no. zsy047 (June 1, 2018): 1–9. *https://doi.org/10.1093/sleep/zsy047.*

Busch, Angela J., Candice L. Schachter, Tom J. Overend, Paul M. Peloso, and Karen A.R. Barber. "Exercise for Fibromyalgia: A Systematic Review." *The Journal of Rheumatology* 35, no. 6, article (June 1, 2008): 1130-1144. *http://www.jrheum.org/content/35/6/1130.abstract*.

Carini, Francesco, Margherita Mazzola, Chiara Fici, Salvatore Palmeri, Massimo Messina, Provvidenza Damiani, and Giovanni Tomasello. "Posture and Posturology, Anatomical and Physiological Profiles: Overview and Current State of Art." *Acta Bio-Medica : Atenei Parmensis* 88, no. 1 (April 28, 2017): 11–16. *https://doi.org/10.23750/abm.v88i1.5309*.

Corazon, Sus Sola, Ulrik Sidenius, Dorthe Varning Poulsen, Marie Christoffersen Gramkow, and Ulrika Karlsson Stigsdotter. "Psycho-Physiological Stress Recovery in Outdoor Nature-Based Interventions: A Systematic Review of the Past Eight Years of Research." *International Journal of Environmental Research and Public Health* 16, no. 10, article no. 1711 (May 16, 2019): 1–21. *https://doi.org/10.3390/ijerph16101711*.

Cramer, Holger, Wolf E. Mehling, Felix J. Saha, Gustav Dobos, and Romy Lauche. "Postural Awareness and Its Relation to Pain: Validation of an Innovative Instrument Measuring Awareness of Body Posture in Patients with Chronic Pain." *BMC Musculoskeletal Disorders* 19: 109 (April 6, 2018): 1–10. *https://doi.org/10.1186/s12891-018-2031-9*.

Gardner, Benjamin, Phillippa Lally, and Jane Wardle. "Making Health Habitual: The Psychology of 'Habit-Formation' and General Practice." *The British Journal of General Practice: The Journal of the Royal College of General Practitioners* 62, no. 605 (December 2012): 664–66. *https://doi.org/10.3399/bjgp12X659466*.

Harvard Health Publishing. "Why Your Annual Check-up Is Still Important to Your Health." *Harvard Health,* Accessed January

19, 2021. *https://www.health.harvard.edu/staying-healthy/why-your-annual-check-up-is-still-important-to-your-health*.

Harvard T. H. Chan School of Public Health. "Vegetables and Fruits." *The Nutrition Source*, September 18, 2012. *https://www.hsph.harvard.edu/nutritionsource/what-should-you-eat/vegetables-and-fruits/*.

Kandola, Aaron, Davy Vancampfort, Matthew Herring, Amanda Rebar, Mats Hallgren, Joseph Firth, and Brendon Stubbs. "Moving to Beat Anxiety: Epidemiology and Therapeutic Issues with Physical Activity for Anxiety." *Current Psychiatry Reports* 20, no. 8 (July 24, 2018): 63. *https://doi.org/10.1007/s11920-018-0923-x*.

Kim, DeokJu, MiLim Cho, YunHee Park, and YeongAe Yang. "Effect of an Exercise Program for Posture Correction on Musculoskeletal Pain." *Journal of Physical Therapy Science* 27, no. 6 (June 2015): 1791–94. *https://doi.org/10.1589/jpts.27.1791*.

Mayo Clinic. "Managing Arthritis Pain." Mayo Clinic. Accessed January 19, 2021. *https://www.mayoclinic.org/diseases-conditions/arthritis/in-depth/arthritis/art-20046440*.

National Heart, Lung, and Blood Institute. "Assessing Your Weight and Health Risk." US Department of Health and Human Services. Accessed January 19, 2021. *https://www.nhlbi.nih.gov/health/educational/lose_wt/risk*.

Patel, Michele L., Christina M. Hopkins, Taylor L. Brooks, and Gary G. Bennett. "Comparing Self-Monitoring Strategies for Weight Loss in a Smartphone App: Randomized Controlled Trial." *JMIR Mhealth Uhealth* 7, no. 2 (February 28, 2019): e12209. *https://doi.org/10.2196/12209*.

Powell, Kenneth E., Amanda E. Paluch, and Steven N. Blair. "Physical Activity for Health: What Kind? How Much? How

Intense? On Top of What?" *Annual Review of Public Health* 32, no. 1 (March 18, 2011): 349–65. *https://doi.org/10.1146/annurev-publhealth-031210-101151.*

Repke, Meredith A., Meredith S. Berry, Lucian G. Conway 3rd, Alexander Metcalf, Reid M. Hensen, and Conor Phelan. "How Does Nature Exposure Make People Healthier?: Evidence for the Role of Impulsivity and Expanded Space Perception." *PloS One* 13, no. 8 (August 22, 2018): e0202246–e0202246. *https://doi.org/10.1371/journal.pone.0202246.*

Seaborne, Robert A., Juliette Strauss, Matthew Cocks, Sam Shepherd, Thomas D. O'Brien, Ken A van Someren, Phillip G Bell, et al. "Human Skeletal Muscle Possesses an Epigenetic Memory of Hypertrophy." *Scientific Reports* 8: article no. 1898 (January 30, 2018): 1–17. *https://doi.org/10.1038/s41598-018-20287-3.*

Silver, Natalie. "Why Does My Weight Fluctuate?" *Healthline*, July 31, 2018. *https://www.healthline.com/health/weight-fluctuation.*

Slavin, Joanne L., and Beate Lloyd. "Health Benefits of Fruits and Vegetables." *Advances in Nutrition (Bethesda, Md.)* 3, no. 4 (July 1, 2012): 506–16. *https://doi.org/10.3945/an.112.002154.*

Teixeira, Pedro J., Eliana V. Carraça, David Markland, Marlene N. Silva, and Richard M. Ryan. "Exercise, Physical Activity, and Self-Determination Theory: A Systematic Review." *The International Journal of Behavioral Nutrition and Physical Activity* 9:78 (June 22, 2012): 1–30. *https://doi.org/10.1186/1479-5868-9-78.*

Worley, Susan L. "The Extraordinary Importance of Sleep: The Detrimental Effects of Inadequate Sleep on Health and Public Safety Drive an Explosion of Sleep Research." *P & T: A Peer-Reviewed Journal for Formulary Management* 43, no. 12 (December 2018): 758–63. *https://pubmed.ncbi.nlm.nih.gov/30559589.*

CHAPTER 4

Contributor, N. T. "Effects of Bedrest 3: Gastrointestinal, Endocrine and Nervous Systems." *Nursing Times* (blog), January 21, 2019. *https://www.nursingtimes.net/clinical-archive/gastroenterology/effects-of-bedrest-3-gastrointestinal-endocrine-and-nervous-systems-21-01-2019/*.

Deslandes, Andrea Camaz. "Exercise and Mental Health: What Did We Learn in the Last 20 Years?" *Frontiers in Psychiatry* 5 (2014): 66. *https://doi.org/10.3389/fpsyt.2014.00066*.

Doherty, Anya, and Anna Forés Miravalles. "Physical Activity and Cognition: Inseparable in the Classroom." *Frontiers in Education* 4: 105 (2019): 1–7. *https://doi.org/10.3389/feduc.2019.00105*.

Erickson, Kirk I., Michelle W. Voss, Ruchika Shaurya Prakash, Chandramallika Basak, Amanda Szabo, Laura Chaddock, Jennifer S. Kim, et al. "Exercise Training Increases Size of Hippocampus and Improves Memory." *Proceedings of the National Academy of Sciences* 108, no. 7 (February 15, 2011): 3017–3022. *https://doi.org/10.1073/pnas.1015950108*.

Guedes, Luana Petruccio Cabral Monteiro, Maria Liz Cunha de Oliveira, and Gustavo de Azevedo Carvalho. "Deleterious Effects of Prolonged Bed Rest on the Body Systems of the Elderly—a Review." *Revista Brasileira de Geriatria e Gerontologia* 21 (2018): 499–506.

Hargens, Alan R., and Laurence Vico. "Long-Duration Bed Rest as an Analog to Microgravity." *Journal of Applied Physiology* 120, no. 8 (February 18, 2016): 891–903. *https://doi.org/10.1152/japplphysiol.00935.2015*.

Howie, Erin K., Jeffrey Schatz, and Russell R. Pate. "Acute Effects of Classroom Exercise Breaks on Executive Function and Math Performance: A Dose-Response Study." *Research Quarterly for*

Exercise and Sport 86, no. 3 (2015): 217–24. *https://doi.org/10.10 80/02701367.2015.1039892.*

NIH Osteoporosis and Related Bone Diseases National Resource Center. "Exercise for Your Bone Health | NIH Osteoporosis and Related Bone Diseases National Resource Center." Accessed January 21, 2021. *https://www.bones.nih.gov/health-info/bone/ bone-health/exercise/exercise-your-bone-health.*

Hallett, Vicky. "Staying Fit Isn't A New Year's Resolution for These Hunter-Gatherers." *NPR.Org*, January 3, 2017. *https://www.npr. org/sections/goatsandsoda/2017/01/03/507562845/staying-fit-isnt-a-new-years-resolution-for-these-hunter-gatherers.*

O'Mara, Shane. *In Praise of Walking: The New Science of How We Walk and Why It's Good for Us.* New York: W. W. Norton & Company, 2020.

Pontzer, H., B. M. Wood, and D. A. Raichlen. "Hunter-Gatherers as Models in Public Health." *Obesity Reviews* 19, no. S1 (December 1, 2018): 24–35. *https://doi.org/10.1111/obr.12785.*

Prince, Stephanie A., Cara G. Elliott, Kyle Scott, Sarah Visintini, and Jennifer L. Reed. "Device-Measured Physical Activity, Sedentary Behaviour and Cardiometabolic Health and Fitness across Occupational Groups: A Systematic Review and Meta-Analysis." *The International Journal of Behavioral Nutrition and Physical Activity* 16: 30 (April 2, 2019): 1–15. *https://doi. org/10.1186/s12966-019-0790-9.*

Raichlen, David A., and Gene E. Alexander. "Adaptive Capacity: An Evolutionary-Neuroscience Model Linking Exercise, Cognition, and Brain Health." *Trends in Neurosciences* 40, no. 7 (July 2017): 408–21. *https://doi.org/10.1016/j.tins.2017.05.001.*

Raichlen, David A., and John D. Polk. "Linking Brains and Brawn: Exercise and the Evolution of Human Neurobiology." *Proceed-*

ings of the Royal Society B: Biological Sciences 280, no. 1750 (January 7, 2013): 1–9. *https://doi.org/10.1098/rspb.2012.2250.*

Raichlen, David A., Herman Pontzer, Theodore W. Zderic, Jacob A. Harris, Audax Z. P. Mabulla, Marc T. Hamilton, and Brian M. Wood. "Sitting, Squatting, and the Evolutionary Biology of Human Inactivity." *Proceedings of the National Academy of Sciences* 117, no. 13 (March 31, 2020): 7115–7121. *https://doi.org/10.1073/pnas.1911868117.*

Ruck for Miles. "Ruck March Shoulder Pain—How to Avoid It". Accessed January 21, 2021. *https://www.ruckformiles.com/guides/ruck-march-shoulder-pain-how-to-avoid-it/.*

Rucking.com. (blog) "Training Program for New Ruckers." November 10, 2018. *https://rucking.com/training-program-for-new-ruckers/.*

Santos-Longhurst, Adrienne. "Average Steps Per Day by Age, Gender, Occupation, and Country." Accessed January 21, 2021. *https://www.healthline.com/health/average-steps-per-day#guidelines.*

Sullivan, Alycia N., and Margie E. Lachman. "Behavior Change with Fitness Technology in Sedentary Adults: A Review of the Evidence for Increasing Physical Activity." *Frontiers in Public Health* 4:289 (January 11, 2017). *https://doi.org/10.3389/fpubh.2016.00289.*

Suwabe, Kazuya, Kyeongho Byun, Kazuki Hyodo, Zachariah M. Reagh, Jared M. Roberts, Akira Matsushita, Kousaku Saotome, et al. "Rapid Stimulation of Human Dentate Gyrus Function with Acute Mild Exercise." *Proceedings of the National Academy of Sciences* 115, no. 41 (October 9, 2018): 10487. *https://doi.org/10.1073/pnas.1805668115.*

Verywell Fit. "Add Confidence and Stability on the Trails with Trekking Poles." Accessed January 21, 2021. *https://www.very-wellfit.com/how-to-use-hiking-and-trekking-poles-for-stability-4145313*.

Verywell Fit. "What Is Nordic Walking?" Accessed January 21, 2021. *https://www.verywellfit.com/nordic-walking-3432907*.

CHAPTER 5

Ailneni, Ravi Charan, Kartheek Reddy Syamala, In-Sop Kim, and Jaejin Hwang. "Influence of the Wearable Posture Correction Sensor on Head and Neck Posture: Sitting and Standing Workstations." *Work* 62, no. 1 (2019): 27–35. *https://doi.org/10.3233/WOR-182839*.

Binstead, Justin T., Akul Munjal, and Matthew Varacallo. "Anatomy, Bony Pelvis and Lower Limb, Calf." In *StatPearls*. Treasure Island (FL): StatPearls Publishing, 2020. *http://www.ncbi.nlm.nih.gov/books/NBK459362/*.

Bordoni, Bruno, and Matthew Varacallo. "Anatomy, Bony Pelvis and Lower Limb, Thigh Quadriceps Muscle." In *StatPearls*. Treasure Island (FL): StatPearls Publishing, 2020. *http://www.ncbi.nlm.nih.gov/books/NBK513334/*.

Carini, Francesco, Margherita Mazzola, Chiara Fici, Salvatore Palmeri, Massimo Messina, Provvidenza Damiani, and Giovanni Tomasello. "Posture and Posturology, Anatomical and Physiological Profiles: Overview and Current State of Art." *Acta Bio-Medica : Atenei Parmensis* 88, no. 1 (April 28, 2017): 11–16. *https://doi.org/10.23750/abm.v88i1.5309*.

Creech, Julie A., and Sabrina Silver. "Shoulder Impingement Syndrome." In *StatPearls*. Treasure Island (FL): StatPearls Publishing, 2020. *http://www.ncbi.nlm.nih.gov/books/NBK554518/*.

Davidovits, P. *Physics in Biology and Medicine*. Complementary Science. Elsevier Science, 2012. *https://books.google.com/books?id=_5G5VRbwCBUC*.

Dynamic Fitness. "Tips for Understanding Muscle Imbalances." Accessed January 22, 2021. *https://dynamicmedicalfitness.com/blog/2019/04/18/tips-for-understanding-muscle-imbalances*.

Elzanie, Adel, and Judith Borger. "Anatomy, Bony Pelvis and Lower Limb, Gluteus Maximus Muscle." In *StatPearls*. Treasure Island (FL): StatPearls Publishing, 2020. *http://www.ncbi.nlm.nih.gov/books/NBK538193/*.

Grgic, Jozo, Alessandro Garofolini, John Orazem, Filip Sabol, Brad J. Schoenfeld, and Zeljko Pedisic. "Effects of Resistance Training on Muscle Size and Strength in Very Elderly Adults: A Systematic Review and Meta-Analysis of Randomized Controlled Trials." *Sports Medicine* 50, no. 11 (November 1, 2020): 1983–99. *https://doi.org/10.1007/s40279-020-01331-7*.

Harvard Health Publishing. "Are Your Hamstrings Working Double Duty?" *Harvard Health*. Accessed January 22, 2021. *https://www.health.harvard.edu/staying-healthy/are-your-hamstrings-working-double-duty*.

Harvard Health Publishing. "Why Good Posture Matters." *Harvard Health*. Accessed January 22, 2021. *https://www.health.harvard.edu/staying-healthy/why-good-posture-matters*.

Healthline. "What Causes Muscle Rigidity?" July 5, 2019. *https://www.healthline.com/health/muscle-rigidity*.

Jenkins, Nathaniel D. M., Amelia A. Miramonti, Ethan C. Hill, Cory M. Smith, Kristen C. Cochrane-Snyman, Terry J. Housh, and Joel T. Cramer. "Greater Neural Adaptations Following High- vs. Low-Load Resistance Training." *Frontiers in Physiology* 8:331 (2017). *https://doi.org/10.3389/fphys.2017.00331*.

Kato, Satoshi, Hideki Murakami, Satoru Demura, Katsuhito Yoshioka, Kazuya Shinmura, Noriaki Yokogawa, Takashi Igarashi, Noritaka Yonezawa, Takaki Shimizu, and Hiroyuki Tsuchiya. "Abdominal Trunk Muscle Weakness and Its Association with Chronic Low Back Pain and Risk of Falling in Older Women." *BMC Musculoskeletal Disorders* 20: 273 (June 3, 2019). *https:// doi.org/10.1186/s12891-019-2655-4.*

Kenhub. "Latissimus Dorsi Muscle." Accessed January 22, 2021. *https://www.kenhub.com/en/library/anatomy/latissimus-dorsi-muscle.*

Laguna Orthopedic Rehabilitation. "Tight Chest Muscles: Why Your Upper Back Is the Key to Their Release." Accessed January 22, 2021. *https://www.lorpt.com/blog/2019/7/24/chest-muscle-tightness-back-related.*

McLeod, Michael, Leigh Breen, D. Lee Hamilton, and Andrew Philp. "Live Strong and Prosper: The Importance of Skeletal Muscle Strength for Healthy Ageing." *Biogerontology* 17, no. 3 (June 2016): 497–510. *https://doi.org/10.1007/s10522-015-9631-7.*

Medical News Today. "Kyphosis: Symptoms, Causes, Exercises, and Treatment." Published January 2, 2019. *https://www.medicalnewstoday.com/articles/324071.*

Medical News Today. "Lordosis: Symptoms, Causes, Treatments, and Exercises," Published June 18, 2020. *https://www.medicalnewstoday.com/articles/lordosis.*

Medical News Today. "Rounded Shoulders: Causes, Risk Factors, Diagnosis, and Exercises," Published July 25, 2017. *https://www.medicalnewstoday.com/articles/318556.*

Medical News Today. "Scoliosis: Treatment, Symptoms, and Causes," March 17, 2020. *https://www.medicalnewstoday.com/articles/190940.*

Medical News Today. "Upper Crossed Syndrome: Causes, Symptoms, and Exercises," Published August 11, 2017. *https://www.medicalnewstoday.com/articles/318897.*

Miniato, Mohammed A., Prashanth Anand, and Matthew Varacallo. "Anatomy, Shoulder and Upper Limb, Shoulder." In *StatPearls.* Treasure Island (FL): StatPearls Publishing, 2020. *http://www.ncbi.nlm.nih.gov/books/NBK536933/.*

Ourieff, Jared, Brent Scheckel, and Amit Agarwal. "Anatomy, Back, Trapezius." In *StatPearls.* Treasure Island (FL): StatPearls Publishing, 2020. *http://www.ncbi.nlm.nih.gov/books/NBK518994/.*

Ransom, Alyssa L., Margaret A. Sinkler, and Shivajee V. Nallamothu. "Anatomy, Bony Pelvis and Lower Limb, Femoral Muscles." In *StatPearls.* Treasure Island (FL): StatPearls Publishing, 2020. *http://www.ncbi.nlm.nih.gov/books/NBK500008/.*

Roubenoff, Ronenn. "Sarcopenia: Effects on Body Composition and Function." *The Journals of Gerontology. Series A, Biological Sciences and Medical Sciences* 58 (December 1, 2003): 1012–17. *https://doi.org/10.1093/gerona/58.11.M1012.*

Sassack, Brett, and Jonathan D. Carrier. "Anatomy, Back, Lumbar Spine." In *StatPearls.* Treasure Island (FL): StatPearls Publishing, 2020. *http://www.ncbi.nlm.nih.gov/books/NBK557616/.*

Seeras, Kevin, Ryan N. Qasawa, Ricky Ju, and Shivana Prakash. "Anatomy, Abdomen and Pelvis, Anterolateral Abdominal Wall." In *StatPearls.* Treasure Island (FL): StatPearls Publishing, 2020. *http://www.ncbi.nlm.nih.gov/books/NBK525975/.*

TrueSports. "Hip Muscle Weakness Can Cause Knee Pain and Injury." True Sports Physical Therapy, January 22, 2020. *https://truesportsphysicaltherapy.com/are-you-neglecting-your-hips.*

Vaughn, Jacob E., and Wayne B. Cohen-Levy. "Anatomy, Bony Pelvis and Lower Limb, Posterior Thigh Muscles." In *StatPearls.* Treasure Island (FL): StatPearls Publishing, 2020. *http://www. ncbi.nlm.nih.gov/books/NBK542215/.*

Vestibular Disorders Association (blog). "The Human Balance System." 2016. Accessed January 22, 2021. *https://vestibular.org/ article/what-is-vestibular/the-human-balance-system/the-hu- man-balance-system-how-do-we-maintain-our-balance/.*

Watson, Steven L., Benjamin K. Weeks, Lisa J. Weis, Amy T. Hard- ing, Sean A. Horan, and Belinda R. Beck. "High-Intensity Resistance and Impact Training Improves Bone Mineral Den- sity and Physical Function in Postmenopausal Women with Osteopenia and Osteoporosis: The LIFTMOR Randomized Controlled Trial." *Journal of Bone and Mineral Research* 33, no. 2 (February 1, 2018): 211–20. *https://doi.org/10.1002/jbmr.3284.*

CHAPTER 6

Cotter, Joshua A., Ait M. Chaudhari, Steve T. Jamison, and Ste- ven T. Devor. "Knee Joint Kinetics in Relation to Commonly Prescribed Squat Loads and Depths." *Journal of Strength and Conditioning Research / National Strength & Conditioning Association* 27, no. 7 (July 2013): 1765–74. *https://doi.org/10.1519/ JSC.0b013e3182773319.*

Gambetta, Vern. "Win the Workout." *HMMR Media* (blog), June 1, 2020. *http://www.hmmrmedia.com/2020/06/win-the-workout/.*

CHAPTER 7

Jay. "Average Vertical Jump: Norms and Scores." *Jumping Uni- verse* (blog), August 18, 2020. *https://jumpinguniverse.com/ average-vertical-jump/.*

Vetrovsky, Tomas, Michal Steffl, Petr Stastny, and James J. Tufano. "The Efficacy and Safety of Lower-Limb Plyometric Training in Older Adults: A Systematic Review." *Sports Medicine* 49, no. 1 (January 1, 2019): 113–31. *https://doi.org/10.1007/s40279-018-1018-x.*

CHAPTER 8

Harvard Health Publishing. "Ask Dr. Rob about Piriformis Syndrome." *Harvard Health.* Accessed January 26, 2021. *https://www.health.harvard.edu/back-pain/ask-dr-rob-about-piriformis-syndrome.*

CHAPTER 9

Deslandes, Andrea Camaz. "Exercise and Mental Health: What Did We Learn in the Last 20 Years?" *Frontiers in Psychiatry* 5: 66 (2014). *https://doi.org/10.3389/fpsyt.2014.00066.*

Fleming, Sara. "From the 1984 Olympics to the Founding of the ISSA". ISSA (blog)." Accessed January 27, 2021. *https://www.issaonline.com/blog/index.cfm/2018/from-the-1984-olympics-to-the-founding-of-the-issa.*

Gardner, Benjamin, Phillippa Lally, and Jane Wardle. "Making Health Habitual: The Psychology of 'habit-Formation' and General Practice." *The British Journal of General Practice : The Journal of the Royal College of General Practitioners* 62, no. 605 (December 2012): 664–66. *https://doi.org/10.3399/bjgp12X659466.*

Hanson, Sarah, and Andy Jones. "Is There Evidence That Walking Groups Have Health Benefits? A Systematic Review and Meta-Analysis." *British Journal of Sports Medicine* 49, no. 11 (June 1, 2015): 710–715. *https://doi.org/10.1136/bjsports-2014-094157.*

Lachman, Margie E., Lewis Lipsitz, James Lubben, Carmen Casta-
neda-Sceppa, and Alan M. Jette. "When Adults Don't Exercise:
Behavioral Strategies to Increase Physical Activity in Sedentary Middle-Aged and Older Adults." *Innovation in Aging* 2,
no. igy007 (April 5, 2018). *https://doi.org/10.1093/geroni/igy007.*

Lee, Harold H., Jessica A. Emerson, and David M. Williams. "The
Exercise–Affect–Adherence Pathway: An Evolutionary Perspective." *Frontiers in Psychology* 7: 1285 (2016). *https://doi.
org/10.3389/fpsyg.2016.01285.*

Murayama, Kou. "The Science of Motivation." American Psychology Association. Accessed January 27, 2021. *https://www.apa.
org/science/about/psa/2018/06/motivation.*

Murayama, Kou, Madoka Matsumoto, Keise Izuma, and Kenji
Matsumoto. "Neural Basis of the Undermining Effect of Monetary Reward on Intrinsic Motivation." *Proceedings of the
National Academy of Sciences* 107, no. 49 (December 7, 2010):
20911–6. *https://doi.org/10.1073/pnas.1013305107.*

Rosa, João P. P., Altay A. L. de Souza, Giscard H. O. de Lima,
Dayane F. Rodrigues, Valdir de Aquino Lemos, Eduardo da
Silva Alves, Sergio Tufik, and Marco T. de Mello. "Motivational
and Evolutionary Aspects of a Physical Exercise Training Pro-
gram: A Longitudinal Study." *Frontiers in Psychology* 6: 648
(May 18, 2015). *https://doi.org/10.3389/fpsyg.2015.00648.*

Teixeira, Pedro J., Eliana V. Carraça, David Markland, Marlene N.
Silva, and Richard M. Ryan. "Exercise, Physical Activity, and
Self-Determination Theory: A Systematic Review." *The International Journal of Behavioral Nutrition and Physical Activity*
9: 78 (June 22, 2012). *https://doi.org/10.1186/1479-5868-9-78.*

Wilson, Kylie, and Darren Brookfield. "Effect of Goal Setting
on Motivation and Adherence in a Six-Week Exercise Program." *International Journal of Sport and Exercise Psychology*

7, no. 1 (January 1, 2009): 89–100. *https://doi.org/10.1080/16121 97X.2009.9671894.*

APPENDIX B

Barber, Dan. *The Third Plate: Field Notes on the Future of Food.* New York: The Penguin Press, 2014.

Crovesy, Louise, Daniele Masterson, and Eliane Lopes Rosado. "Profile of the Gut Microbiota of Adults with Obesity: A Systematic Review." *European Journal of Clinical Nutrition* 74, no. 9 (September 1, 2020): 1251–62. *https://doi.org/10.1038/s41430-020-0607-6.*

Garaulet, M., P. Gómez-Abellán, J. J. Alburquerque-Béjar, Y-C Lee, J. M. Ordovás, and F. A. J. L. Scheer. "Timing of Food Intake Predicts Weight Loss Effectiveness." *International Journal of Obesity* 37, no. 4 (April 1, 2013): 604–11. *https://doi.org/10.1038/ ijo.2012.229.*

Glenn, Jordan M, Erica N. Madero, and Nick T. Bott. "Dietary Protein and Amino Acid Intake: Links to the Maintenance of Cognitive Health." *Nutrients* 11, no. 6, article no. 1315 (June 12, 2019). *https://doi.org/10.3390/nu11061315.*

Harvard Health Publishing. "Know the Facts about Fats." *Harvard Health.* Accessed January 31, 2021. *https://www.health.harvard. edu/staying-healthy/know-the-facts-about-fats.*

Harvard Health Publishing. "Why Weight Matters When It Comes to Joint Pain." *Harvard Health.* Accessed January 27, 2021. *https://www.health.harvard.edu/pain/why-weight-matters-when-it-comes-to-joint-pain.*

Healthline. "What Are the Key Functions of Carbohydrates?" Published November 9, 2017. *https://www.healthline.com/nutrition/ carbohydrate-functions.*

Kreher, Jeffrey B., and Jennifer B. Schwartz. "Overtraining Syndrome: A Practical Guide." *Sports Health* 4, no. 2 (March 2012): 128–38. *https://doi.org/10.1177/1941738111434406*.

Leulier, François, Lesley T. MacNeil, Won-jae Lee, John F. Rawls, Patrice D. Cani, Martin Schwarzer, Liping Zhao, and Stephen J. Simpson. "Integrative Physiology: At the Crossroads of Nutrition, Microbiota, Animal Physiology, and Human Health." *Cell Metabolism* 25, no. 3 (March 7, 2017): 522–34. *https://doi.org/10.1016/j.cmet.2017.02.001*.

Mayo Clinic. "Trans Fat: Double Trouble for Your Heart." Accessed January 30, 2021. *https://www.mayoclinic.org/diseases-conditions/high-blood-cholesterol/in-depth/trans-fat/art-20046114*.

Paoli, Antonio, Grant Tinsley, Antonino Bianco, and Tatiana Moro. "The Influence of Meal Frequency and Timing on Health in Humans: The Role of Fasting." *Nutrients* 11, no. 4, article no. 719 (March 28, 2019): 7–9. *https://doi.org/10.3390/nu11040719*.

Pontzer, H., B. M. Wood, and D. A. Raichlen. "Hunter-Gatherers as Models in Public Health." *Obesity Reviews* 19, no. S1 (December 1, 2018): 24–35. *https://doi.org/10.1111/obr.12785*.

Pontzer, Herman. "Evolved to Exercise." *Scientific American*, January 2019.

Pontzer, Herman. "The Crown Joules: Energetics, Ecology, and Evolution in Humans and Other Primates." *Evolutionary Anthropology: Issues, News, and Reviews* 26, no. 1 (January 1, 2017): 12–24. *https://doi.org/10.1002/evan.21513*.

Pontzer, Herman, Ramon Durazo-Arvizu, Lara R. Dugas, Jacob Plange-Rhule, Pascal Bovet, Terrence E. Forrester, Estelle V. Lambert, Richard S. Cooper, Dale A. Schoeller, and Amy Luke. "Constrained Total Energy Expenditure and Metabolic Adaptation to Physical Activity in Adult Humans." *Current Biology:*

CB 26, no. 3 (February 8, 2016): 410–17. *https://doi.org/10.1016/j. cub.2015.12.046.*

Rodriguez, Nancy R. "Introduction to Protein Summit 2.0: Continued Exploration of the Impact of High-Quality Protein on Optimal Health." *The American Journal of Clinical Nutrition* 101, no. 6 (June 1, 2015): 1317S–1319S. *https://doi.org/10.3945/ ajcn.114.083980.*

Schatzker, Mark. *The Dorito Effect: The Surprising New Truth About Food and Flavor.* New York: Simon and Schuster Paperbacks, 2015.

US Department of Agriculture. "MyPlate." Accessed January 31, 2021. *https://www.myplate.gov/.*

Valenzuela, Pedro L., Alejandro Santos-Lozano, Alberto Torres Barrán, Pablo Fernández-Navarro, Adrián Castillo-García, Luis M. Ruilope, David Ríos Insua, José M. Ordovas, Victoria Ley, and Alejandro Lucia. "Joint Association of Physical Activity and Body Mass Index with Cardiovascular Risk: A Nationwide Population-Based Cross-Sectional Study." *European Journal of Preventive Cardiology*, no. zwaa151 (January 22, 2021). *https://doi.org/10.1093/eurjpc/zwaa151.*

Webb, Denise. "Protein for Fitness: Age Demands Greater Protein Needs." Magazine. *Today's Dietician*, April 2015. *https://www. todaysdietitian.com/newarchives/040715p16.shtml.*

Westerterp, K. R. "Control of Energy Expenditure in Humans." *European Journal of Clinical Nutrition* 71, no. 3 (March 1, 2017): 340–44. *https://doi.org/10.1038/ejcn.2016.237.*

Westerterp, Klaas R. "Exercise, Energy Balance and Body Composition." *European Journal of Clinical Nutrition* 72, no. 9 (September 2018): 1246–50. *https://doi.org/10.1038/s41430-018-0180-4.*

Yanai, Hidekatsu. "Nutrition for Sarcopenia." *Journal of Clinical Medicine Research* 7, no. 12 (December 2015): 926–31. *https://doi.org/10.14740/jocmr2361w.*

Made in the USA
Columbia, SC
12 May 2021